SHE HIK

Being an Occupational Therapist, I am passionate about improving and enhancing both the mind and body through functional movement and daily tasks. For an able-bodied person, walking is a fundamental activity that can promote and advance holistic health and well-being.

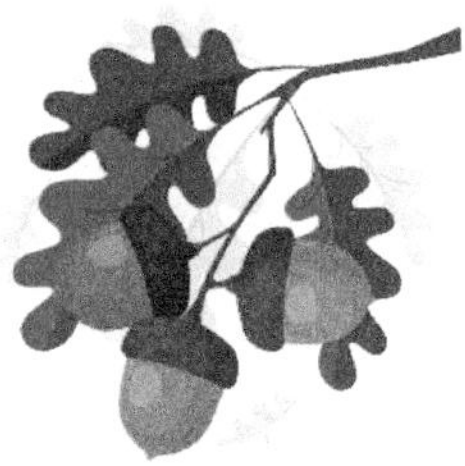

'DON'T DIE WITH MUSIC INSIDE YOU'

(Wayne Dyer)

When you have something beautiful still to give, get it out there for the world to share.

CONTENTS

Introduction	*Page............................4-5*
Planning/Itinerary	*Page............................6-9*
Training	*Page............................10 - 11*
Boots	*Page............................12 - 15*
Footcare	*Page............................16 - 17*
Walking Poles	*Page............................18 - 19*
Cows	*Page............................20 - 21*
Farm Dogs	*Page............................22 - 23*
Toilets	*Page............................24 - 25*
Day Hike Packing List	*Page............................26 - 29*
Overnight Packing List	*Page............................30 - 32*
My 10 Essential Items	*Page............................33*
Post-Hike	*Page............................34 - 35*
Post-Hike Stretches	*Page............................36 - 37*
Safety	*Page............................38 - 39*
Fellow Hikers	*Page............................40*
Dining Alone	*Page............................41 - 42*
Why Do We Walk?	*Page............................43 – 45*
Mind & Soul	*Page............................46 - 47*
Forest Bathing	*Page............................48*
Smile	*Page............................49 - 50*
My Walking Heroes	*Page............................51 - 52*

My Walking Influences *Page.............................53 - 54*

Enjoy *Page.............................55*

My Walking Adventures *Page.............................56 - 106*

Acknowledgements *Page............................107 - 108*

References / Further Reading *Page............................109*

INTRODUCTION

Times are changing.... there is no longer such a taboo around solo female hikers. In fact, in my experience, there seems to be a lot of respect and awe out there for us laced-up lonesome ladies.

Remember, however, that there is a difference between being 'lonely' and being 'alone'.

Hiking alone is a choice, and one made for many reasons. For me, walking alone is empowering and liberating; it allows me to get close and in touch with nature and the earth around me whilst having the space and time to be with my thoughts.

Being in the sunlight plays a vital role in regulating hormones and neurotransmitters in the brain, which heightens feelings of well-being, energy and happiness.

The outdoors is an arena of tranquillity that allows me to balance my mind, without distraction, whilst also executing and achieving a challenge I've set for myself.

By no means is this book meant to belittle the challenges solo male hikers may have; I can only speak from my own experiences as a woman and the challenges I've encountered in the hope it may help or encourage others teetering on the edge of going out alone.

As a solo female hiker it can be daunting and unnerving when you decide to start out walking alone, but the benefits hugely outweigh these fears. There is so much to be gained on a mental, spiritual and mindful level (not to mention the physical advantages) that you cannot always experience when hiking with others.

I hope that you ladies (and any gentlemen that may be reading this) find some answers and some pearls of wisdom in this book to move you towards your solo hiking liberation.

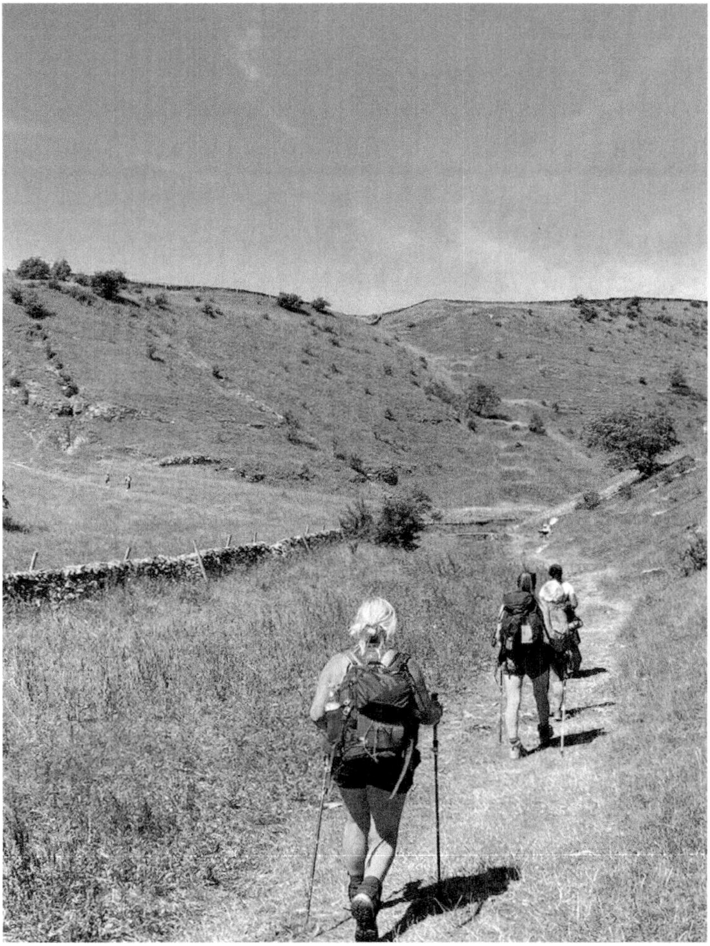

PLANNING/ITINERARY

This part is an absolute must. As my Girl Guide leader (Brown Owl) would say: 'Be Prepared'. This is the most pivotal part of any successful adventure – unless, of course, you're a person who doesn't worry and who excels at living life on the edge (in which case, you probably don't need this book).

When hiking with others, there can be a sense of thrill in winging it, maybe not knowing – or even caring – where you're going to end up that night. It can be exciting and fun.

However, for me, when hiking and travelling alone, I like and need to know exactly what I'm doing and where I'm heading. I like to know where I'm going to stay that night (if camping), or a time frame for when I'll get home. This eliminates some of the anxiety and leaves more space for enjoyment.

There are extreme advantages to being prepared in terms of your safety. For instance, you don't want to be out after dark if you're not planning to. This will bring you a whole host of other challenges.

- *Weather* – Check the weather (on various sites) to see what to expect. This way you can pack accordingly and adjust your route/plans if required.
- *Clothing* – With the above being said, you never quite know what the weather will throw at you. It is best to be prepared for all eventualities to ensure a

more pleasurable adventure. They say there's no such thing as bad weather… just bad clothing!

- *Distance* – This will depend on the terrain and the speed you are walking. I like to allow three miles an hour on the flat and two miles an hour on hills (and add on stoppage time).
  It is much better to underestimate your distance per hour than overestimate. You can always tag some extra stomping on at the end if you finish early (or you could resign to the pub!).
- *Breaks* – Allow adequate rest stops. Regular stops will allow you time off your feet and will give your body a chance to recharge and recuperate.
  I like to take my boots off at regular stops, air my feet, inspect them for damage, and give them some TLC. This is also a good time to put on fresh, dry socks (wet ones can be hung on the back of your pack to dry and reuse later if needed).
- *Maps* – Do not leave the house without some form of map. Even if you're walking locally and think you know where you're going, with a map you can explore other paths and tracks you may find and make it a real adventure.
  I just LOVE the OS App. This allows me to plot and plan my route beforehand, get an estimated mileage and, with the GPS running, it will tell me where I am on the route at all times. This has been invaluable in putting me back on the path when I've got lost or finding an alternative route if one is blocked (or if it contains fields of not-so-friendly livestock).

- *Chargers* - Ensure your phone is fully charged and that you have a charging device (battery pack, bank or solar charger) with you. Using some apps will drain your battery and you need to be sure you can contact help if needed.
- *Trackers* – Ensure someone knows where you're planning to go and your estimated time of return. Check in with someone when you get home or, if possible, let someone keep an eye on you with a tracker.
- *Start* - If you're not starting your hike from your doorstep, plan how you're going to reach the starting point (bus, train, taxi etc.) and allow for this in your time schedule. Check public transport times and delays prior to travel to avoid disruption.
- *Contacts* - If you're doing a multi-day hike, make sure you have a paper copy of your itinerary (in case your phone dies or gets lost). Have the contacts of the places you intend to stay and ensure that they're expecting you with a rough ETA. Confirm your bookings prior to departure to avoid any panic, stress or disappointment on arrival.
- *Rest days* - If on a multi-day hike, ensure you factor in some rest time. Whether they be whole days or half days, they will be invaluable when your feet are sore and you need some respite. This will also allow you to check out local towns/points of interest and make your adventure more varied and memorable.
- *Water* - Consider your water replenishment. If you're likely to need more water than you're able to carry, look on the map and mark places – cafes,

pubs etc. – on your route where you can refill. The same goes for food. If you cannot carry the amount you need for your entire trip, then pre-plan places where you can restock.
Water purification tablets take up little space. If you're planning to go off-grid, where there will be natural water sources available, this would be a sensible thing to pack.

- *Supplies* - When I did the Pennine Way I was unsure where I would find food/supplies. So, I sent forward packages of dried foods, plasters, etc. to various campsites I'd booked into before I left – and hey presto... they were there waiting for me at each destination. Be sure to add a little treat to each pack (chocolate, face mask, foot mask, etc.). This is not only an incentive to get there but an absolute pick-me-up when you most need it.

TRAINING

Part of the preparation for a successful hike is the training, ensuring you're fit enough to complete the route you have planned. For example, it would be unwise to plan a 20-mile walk if you've only ever walked two or three miles. That's not to say you wouldn't achieve it, but you may not enjoy it much and your body may suffer afterwards.

Training will allow you to identify any niggles, issues and re-thinks you may need to ensure you have a successful adventure.

When I was training for the Pennine Way I totally overestimated the amount of weight I could carry. I went out with the gear I was intending to take on my trip and very soon realised I either needed to reduce the load (quite dramatically) or reduce the daily mileage, as otherwise it was going to end in tears....big fat tears, just as that first day of training did, resulting in me having to call my dad to come and pick me up!

- *Maps* – If you're using an OS map, ensure you have plotted your route and are able to read a map (I know... sounds obvious).
- *Trials* – Do some trial walks. Plot your route and go out and execute it. Keep an eye on the map for landmarks and roads/tracks to ensure you stay on course.
- *Navigation* – If you're required to use a compass to successfully complete your hike, take some tutorials

and then get outdoors and practise. At the very least, ensure you can find North!

- *OS* - I cannot advocate enough the use of the OS App. I know some say this is cheating, but for a woman out there on her own, this by far gives me my biggest peace of mind. And I get lost way less now than I did before I had this app! This is by no means meant to replace a paper map as you cannot rely solely on technology, but it does add another tool to your box.
- *Terrain* – When training, choose a terrain that is similar to that of your planned hike (if possible). This has proved tricky for me over the years, living in Norfolk.
- *Clothing* – Dress appropriately for the foreseen weather. Layers are a great idea as you can add and take away as your body or the external temperature changes. Also, light layers will dry quicker when wet and, if you're hiking over a period of days, you can alternate which ones are closer to your sweaty skin. Train with the clothes you intend to wear (including underwear) to eliminate any potential discomfort or chafing.

BOOTS

Your hiking boots or shoes are the single most important piece of kit you'll need. NEVER start a long hike in a new pair of boots without breaking them in first. It will only bring you misery!

- *Size* – If you're buying new boots/shoes, ensure you try them on in the shop and walk around in them for a bit too. The recommendation is to buy boots between half and a full size larger than your feet to allow for thick socks, double-layered socks, and swelling.
  When you get them home, wear them around indoors as much as possible to allow your feet to mould into them. This will also allow you time to ensure they are right for you and to return them if needed.
  If you plan to walk on rough terrain or have particular weaknesses in your ankles, be sure to consider boots with good ankle support.
  Ensure the width is adequate – particularly if you have wide feet. I gravitate towards buying men's shoes as these tend to be wider and I find them more comfortable.
- *Laces* – Ensure you have good laces. I find that the cylinder-type laces can slip and then I spend all day retying them. Instead, I like to use flat laces and double-tie them. Ensuring the laces are tight enough can be key to preventing your feet from slipping and therefore chafing in the boot. There

are numerous tutorials you can access online on how to lace up your boots correctly.
Always carry a spare pair of laces, as you'll be a bit stuck if one breaks. You also never know where a spare lace will come in handy!

- *Insoles* – I like to carry a spare pair of insoles with me, as when the soles of my feet feel sore and on fire (or my boots are wet), I find changing the insole and adding more cushioning helps. Play around with this prior to your hike to see what works for you.
- *Gaiters* – I tend to wear ankle gaiters on all my walks these days. They prevent dust and stones from getting into my boots so I don't need to stop so often to take them off and shake them out. They will also prevent (to some degree) rain from getting into your boots and making them wet on the inside, as well as protecting your boots and legs when walking through long grass and nettles.
- *Hot spots* – Whenever you recognise a hot spot on your foot, it is important to stop and address it. Strap it, plaster it, or change your socks if they're causing friction, but don't leave it; it will only get worse and then become a misery.
- *Drying your boots* – Be sure to dry your boots out after each hike (especially if you're hiking in them the next day). Some campsites provide drying rooms. If not, try the airing cupboard, place them beside a radiator, or stuff newspaper into them and open them up to the air. If your boots are wet on the inside when you need to put them on again, try

placing large sandwich bags or doggy poo bags on each foot between two pairs of socks. This will form a barrier between your feet and the wet boots and keep them dry and snug.

I do have some waterproof socks – these are great for keeping your feet dry from the dampness of your boot, but they also cause your feet to sweat so they become wet anyway. They are most effective in cold weather when your boots are wet.

- *Spare shoes* – If you're able to, carry a spare pair of lightweight shoes with you (sandals, plimsols etc.). If you need your boots the next day, your feet will be grateful to be out of them and it will give them time to dry.

  They will also come in handy if you develop blisters that become unbearable to walk on, if your boots get saturated, or if you just need to get your boots off at the end of your hike.
- *Dry feet* - If you find yourself needing to cross streams/rivers and are likely to end up with wet boots, don't do it. Instead, take your boots off and walk through in bare feet. Or, if you have some large dry bags, stick these over your boots. You and your feet will be eternally thankful to have dry boots later on the walk and in the following days.

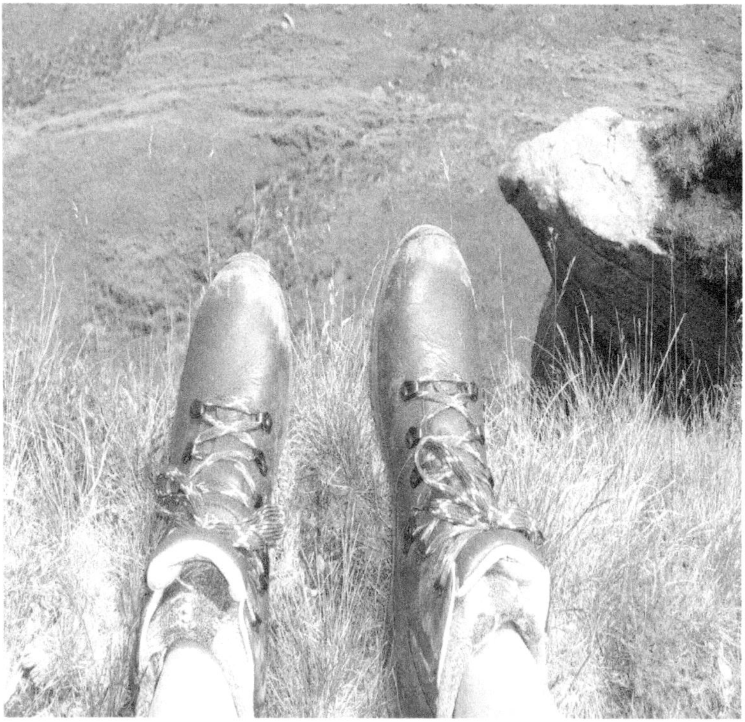

FOOTCARE

Footcare is so, so important before, during, and after your hike. Look after your feet and they will look after you!

- *Prep hike* – Some people believe you need to harden your feet up before embarking on a long hike. In the past, I've tried surgical spirit and even soaking my feet in tea. I can't say either method was very effective for me, but I know others that have found it so; it may be worth a try if you have soft, delicate tootsies.
- *Blisters* – If you're unfortunate enough to suffer from blisters, they will likely be the biggest obstacle you'll have. The key is to identify vulnerable areas before they become too much of an issue. If you know there are areas of your feet that will bother you, tape or plaster them up before setting off.
  I use toe sleeves on my little toes – which often flare up – and this seems to help. Later on in a hike, I also use zinc tape to wrap the ball of my foot as I know this can become a problem for me. If you think taping your feet is for you, look up a YouTube tutorial on the most effective method.
  Popping blisters is a controversial subject. It can be painful walking on a blister full of fluid. If possible, I make a (very small) pinprick to release the fluid, use antiseptic cream, and then cover it well. The risk of popping it mid-hike is that the roof of the blister will come away, exposing very raw skin underneath. This can be excruciatingly painful!

I would advise you not to rip off plasters (especially blister plasters) in the bath after your walk (unless, of course, they are hanging off). I've done this many times, taking the top layer of skin with it and leaving it sore and exposed for days.

- *Friction* – I use a skin shield (foot lubrication) on my feet before putting my socks on. This helps reduce the friction in the boot/shoe and prevent chafing. I re-apply this every few miles or when changing my socks.
  I know others that like to use talc, as this has a different approach of keeping the foot dry to prevent the skin from becoming soft and tearing.
  It is widely suggested that two pairs of socks should be used to reduce friction. If you decide to do this, I suggest using a thin (trainer-type) sock underneath and then a more robust walking sock over the top.
  You can buy double-layered socks that offer the same principle. I often find this effective during long hikes.
- *Socks* – If you can, invest in some good wick away walking socks. These are designed to keep your feet dryer and less prone to blisters.
  Always carry spare socks and dry them in between – you never know when you may need to re-use them!

WALKING POLES

Besides boots, these are one of the most essential and precious items on my hiking kit list. They're definitely not everyone's preference, though, and you can feel a bit of a goof, especially when tapping away on a flat road!

However, when it's late in the day and your legs are tired, or you have achy hips and knees (as I generally do these days), they're a lifeline in terms of getting me home.

TIP – Try not to touch electric fences with them... not much fun!

- *Oedematous hands* – Anyone that has carried out a day hike (without poles) will be familiar with the 'sausage fingers'. This occurs when walking for a period of time with your hands by your side. When walking with poles, this doesn't happen as your hands are elevated and moving.
  Using poles also gives your upper body some movement, which is good for circulation and removing oedema (and you burn more calories as you're working the upper muscle groups too – win-win).
- *Balance* – If you have poor balance, poles are great for steadying yourself on uneven ground and keeping you upright.
  If you're on boggy ground, you can place them before your step to judge the depth of a bog or puddle and to ensure the ground is solid and not bottomless.

- *Nettles* – Poles are a great way to hold back nettles and brambles to clear the path ahead of you.
- *Cattle* – If you're caught in a confrontation with a cow or bull (or any type of animal, for that matter) you can gently use your poles to shoo them out of the way. This will keep them an additional arm's length from you.

Walking poles are generally lightweight and easy to store, either inside or on the outside of your rucksack. It's a personal choice but they get the thumbs up from me.

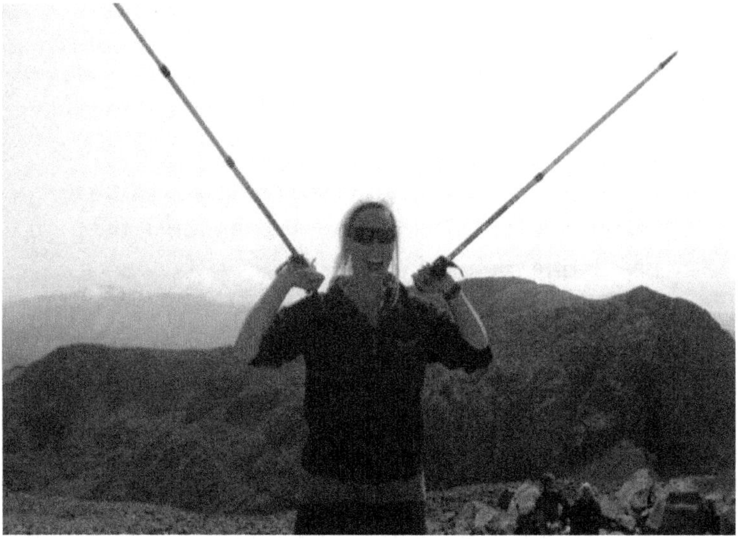

Now, this is a subject very close to my heart. I cannot tell you the number of times I've been chased through fields by cows and cattle, or the number of ditches and fences I've vaulted to avoid being trampled into the earth.

I have fallen on the mercy of many farmers to escort me through or around their livestock when I've been in trouble and very close to hysteria.

- Firstly, reccy every field before entering. Figure out the location of your exit on the other side of the field, keep the border in view at all times and, if necessary, skirt around the edges where you can jump a fence or wall to safety. Don't leave yourself exposed in the middle of a field.
- Check out if the animals are bulls or cows and if they have any young with them. Bulls have never given me as much trouble as cows have when they're with their young (understandably, they are protecting their babies).
- Give them a wide berth and the respect they deserve. Remember, you're in their home space.
- Take deep breaths and keep yourself calm. Sing a little song or hum a tune (or as I often do, chat to them). They will pick up on your anxiety and fear, which can put them on edge.
- Make noise and make yourself seen and heard so as not to startle them. I tend to hang around the gate making noise until they spot me to see what their reaction is. If they put their heads back down and

carry on eating, or don't even get up, then you're probably fine to make your move.

- This is a wimpy thing to do but, if there are other people around you, allow them to go first and hang back and watch... if they make it through alive, you'll likely be OK.
- Keep your walking poles (if you have them – if not, find a big stick) at hand. These can be useful to keep some distance between you and them, if needed.
- If they start to get interested and congregate in your direction, it may be wise to consult the map and see if you can find an alternative route.
- If (heaven forbid) you end up being chased, run in a zig-zag direction as cows cannot stop and turn as fast as you can (this is easy to say, but when you have a stampede behind you, your first instinct is to just flipping RUN).
- Once you've made it through the field, check to see if others are behind you. If so, use your whistle and signal them to take a wide berth.

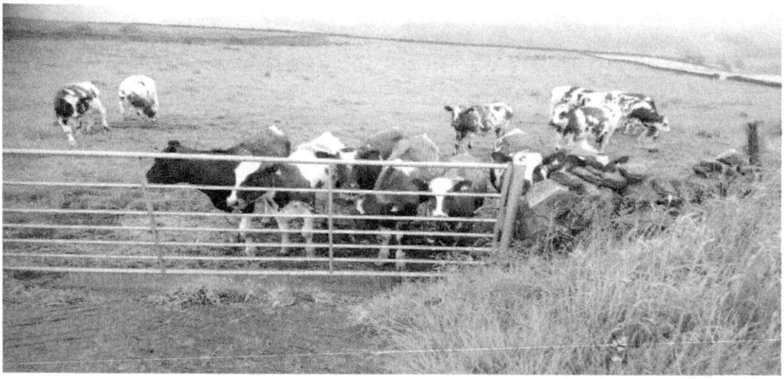

FARM DOGS

Farm dogs are probably your biggest threat when walking through farmyards and any land belonging to farmhouses (that said, I have been held hostage by a pheasant before... but that is a story for another time). I think you only need one encounter of being chased by a territorial farm dog to feel cautious when entering any form of farm estate for the rest of your life. Well, this has very much been my experience.

- Before entering through any gates into the property/yard, take a good scan of the area, figure out your route and, if you can, keep your eye on the next gate/fence available to you to jump over if necessary.
- Make noise to draw attention to yourself prior to going through the gate, so you have the safety of the gate between you should you need it.
- Carry your poles; these can be vital in keeping the animal away from you.
- ALWAYS stick to the path. Follow the arrows (if there are any, that is) that are meant for walkers. Responsible farmers should not place their aggressive animals in your path.
- If you are confronted by a dog and cannot easily escape, then stand still. Keep your poles at length and call for help. Walk slowly towards your nearest exit or barrier.
- I have since purchased an animal deterrent spray (citronella, as pepper spray is illegal in the UK). If nothing else, it gives me peace of mind to have

something I can spray at an animal (or bird, as the pheasant incident is what spurred me to purchase this) to buy myself time to run! I'm not sure how effective this would be on a cow or even another human, but I would give it a go if needed.

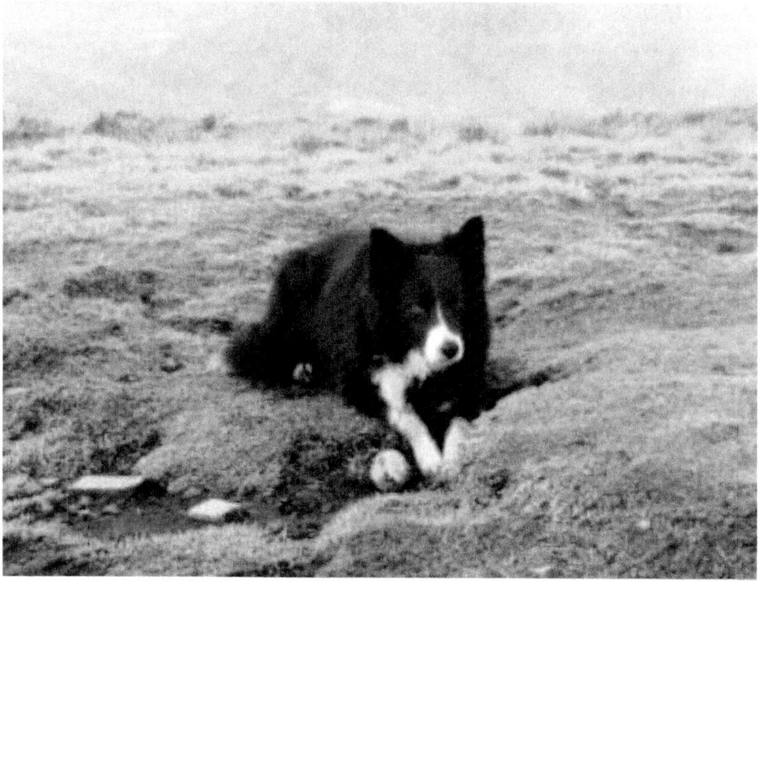

TOILETS

Oh yes, the good old subject of toileting. As a female, it is somewhat more challenging to have a quick pee stop than it is for a gentleman. With the added danger of not having a buddy to watch your back, this is often a daunting (but very necessary) procedure.

That said, many a time I have much preferred to toilet in nature than in some of the putrid, disgusting, and – quite frankly – inhumane public toilet facilities that are out there (I think Nepal is currently holding the torch on this one).

I have, in the past, tried the Shewee. For me, this wasn't too successful, and I found it was just as quick (if not quicker) and much less hassle to just squat in nature than mess around with this device. But I know it works for some, so it may be something to try.

- Try to use a section of the path where you have a clear line of vision in both directions for some way. This will buy you time to do the business (obviously, away from any water sources).
- Move off the path once the way is clear to find your preferred squat site. Listen hard to ensure you're alone before dropping your drawers.
- I have, in the past, placed a hi-vis object on the opposite side and a few metres along the path to detract focus from myself in case someone does come by – in particular, bikes, which you will have no warning about and which will result in you becoming frozen in action.

- Always carry toilet paper and dog poop bags if it's not possible to bury your business/tissues safely and discreetly. I once had to use a teabag (albeit a green teabag!) instead of a tissue, as this was all I had in my pocket and I was up a mountain above the treeline, where there was little greenery. Foliage can work well, but opt for the soft mossy types as opposed to the prickly or waxy ones.
- Some people carry trowels on long walks. This depends on your preference and on your ability to carry additional weight.

As a woman, you may have monthly lady concerns. Don't let this stop you from getting out there. Be sure to carry supplies, tissues, wipes, and bags for discarding waste and you'll be just fine.

If you suffer with cramps and pains, take the appropriate pain relief before and during your hike, and even consider heat patches that you can tuck under your waistband.

The 'moon cup' may also be something worth considering. I've not used this myself so cannot comment, but I know of other outdoor ladies who would highly recommend it.

DAY HIKE PACKING LIST

My current pack is 35 litres. I also have a 25-litre one for short day walks and a 65-litre one for self-sufficient overnight treks.

After each hike, I tend to leave my rucksack packed with the basic essentials. However, this can be dangerous as, in the past, I've forgotten to restock certain items such as plasters and pain relief and have been caught out.

If you're new to hiking and have not yet bought yourself an adequate rucksack, I would suggest you consider one that has an AirZone back (to reduce sweating), padded adjustable straps (for comfort and to reduce chafing), a substantial waist strap that doesn't cut into you, pockets for easy access to essential snacks and your phone etc., separate inside pockets to keep items safe and dry, and a detachable rain cover (this doubles up nicely as something to sit on when the ground is wet).

- *Water* – The amount depends on the weather and the length of your walk.
- *Food/snacks* – High-energy snacks (cereal bars, jelly babies, nuts, dried fruit, Kendal Mint Cake), though again it depends on the amount of time you're planning to be out for.
- *Whistle* (many packs have these built in these days).
- *Compass* (take a few lessons and do some practice runs before heading out (YouTube has some great tutorials).

- *Maps* - Ensure you have maps to cover the entire area you intend to walk. A waterproof map cover is suggested if you don't have the waterproof version.
- *Phone App* – I subscribe to the OS Maps app, which I find beyond worth it, especially when lost.
- *Chargers/charging bank/solar charger* (don't forget the lead).
- *Walking poles* (lightweight and collapsible so you can attach to your pack when not using).
- *Lightweight poncho/waterproofs* (a poncho is great for light showers as you can just throw it over yourself and your pack without having to faff around. However, if it is settled rain you would be better with a proper waterproof coat (with a mesh inner lining, if possible, for ventilation), waterproof trousers, and a backpack cover.
- *Gaiters* – I won't go out now without them. Not only do they prevent the rain from entering the top of your boots, but they also prevent all the dust, grit, and stones from getting in too. I find the ankle ones are sufficient most of the time.
- *First Aid Kit* – For me, this comprises plasters (standard, moleskins, and blister varieties), pain killers, strapping tape, nail scissors, antibacterial gel/wipes, antiseptic cream, bug spray (miniature one), antihistamines, safety pins, talc (I put a little into a plastic sandwich bag to save space and weight – it does look a little suspicious though!), anti-chafing gel/Vaseline, and Imodium. It seems like a long list but you only need to take a few of

each item (not the full boxes). This will keep the space and weight down.

- *Plastic bag* – For wet items of clothing.
- *Sunscreen* (I take a miniature travel one).
- *Space blanket* – You never know when you or someone you meet may need it. It's small, compact, and lightweight, and it could prove to be your most vital piece of kit.
- *Sunglasses.*
- *Sun hat/cap* – I find a cap very useful as it can be used for a sunshade and also to keep the rain or wind from your face/eyes.
- *Head torch* (with spare batteries) – You may not plan to be out after dark but if you get lost, this will be invaluable.
- *Hi-vis vest.*
- *Water purification tablets* (if you run out of water and need to drink from a natural water source).
- *Spare socks* – These can also be used as mittens if it's colder than expected and you don't have any gloves.
- *Tissues* – For toileting needs, and runny noses.
- *Trowel* – If you have the space and feel it will be necessary.
- *Spare laces*
- *Lightweight sandals/plimsols* – I would only take these on a substantial hike. However, they could come in handy if your boots break, get saturated, or even lost (we've all seen that random boot and wondered… how??). Also, they're great to change

into at the end of a walk if you're not heading straight home.

- *Sarong* – I know this sounds odd but, for me, this item has come in useful time and time again. It is a versatile piece of kit that is lightweight and can be used as a towel, bandage, headcover, knee strap, blanket to sit on... its functions are endless.
- *Bandana* – This has come in so, so handy. I have used mine as a sunhat, neck warmer, sweatband, and drippy nose wiper, and it can also be placed on your thigh to prevent chafing if your trousers are wet or rubbing.
- *Cash* – It's always useful to have some cash in case you need to pay for a taxi or bus, or if you need to purchase something from a shop that doesn't accept card payments.
- *Taxi* - Always have a local taxi firm number on you in the event you get lost or injured, or if you find yourself running out of daylight and need to call for a lift.

OVERNIGHT PACKING LIST

If I'm hiking and camping overnight, and carrying all my gear, I'll take my larger, 65 litre backpack. I try not to pack it any heavier than 15kg, but this depends on the amount of water I need to carry.

Additional items to those stated in the day packing list might include:

- *Dry bags* - to keep items separate in case they get wet.
- *Penknife.*
- *Small towel* (quick drying).
- *Toothbrush/toothpaste* (travel size).
- *Soap bar* - that can be used for body and hair (or sachet shampoo to save space).
- *Earplugs* – Personally, I'd rather not hear what's going on outside my tent… if it's gonna get me, it's gonna get me!
- *Padlock* – This is a bizarre item to pack, I know… However, if nothing else it works as a deterrent to intruders, and it will buy me some time to find the penknife (haha).
- *Tent* – I have a small, lightweight two-man tent (I get too claustrophobic in the one-man ones) and I need to have enough headroom to sit upright.
- *Sleeping bag* – A lightweight three-season with a silk liner for colder times of the year.
- *Roll mat* – Lightweight and inflatable.
- *Air pillow.*
- *Gas burner* – With foldable and detachable stove.

- *Matches/lighter* (keep in a separate compartment and keep dry).
- *Mess tin* – To save space, I use this both to boil water and to eat out of.
- *Spork.*
- *Lightweight cup.*
- *Small sponge* - for washing up.
- *Dehydrated food packs* – These are lightweight, nutritionally balanced, and only require hot water to make – plus, you can eat out of the bag so there's no washing up!
- *Hydration/Camel pack* – I tend to use this overnight to save space.
- *Woolly hat* – You will lose most of your body heat through your head.
- *Gloves* (if expecting cold weather).
- *Layers* – Thin, lightweight and breathable layers that can be combined for warmth.
- Something dry and close to the skin to sleep in (e.g. leggings and a thermal top).
- *Underwear*
- *Spare socks* – These are not only used for the obvious (on your feet) but, as mentioned before, they can be used on your hands if you don't have gloves. I also use them on my shoulders – placing them under the pack straps if they're rubbing on my skin – especially in warm weather when you have fewer layers on.
- *Non-thermal flask* – You can use this to carry water by day, and at night as a hot water bottle (hence

non-thermal). Just place a sock over it (preferably a clean one) to keep nice and toasty.

- *Duct tape* – The versatile tape that can be used in many unforeseen situations i.e patching your tent. To save space I wrap this around my gas cannister instead of carrying the whole reel.
- TOP TIP – *Laundry sheets* – These are fabulous at keeping all the wet and dirty items in your pack smelling fresh. Wrap your clothes in them and even place a few inside your sleeping bag to kid yourself that you're sleeping under fresh clean sheets!

MY 10 ESSENTIAL ITEMS

- Phone/chargers
- OS Maps/app (GPS)
- Walking poles
- Water
- Waterproofs
- First aid kit
- High energy snacks
- Spare socks
- Foil blanket
- Sarong/bandana (my versatile piece of kit)

POST-HIKE

It's very important to take care of your feet and your body even after you've finished your hike. Your body has worked hard for you, and now you need to show it some gratitude and respect.

- *Hydration* – Be sure to hydrate well. I often seem to crave cold milk after a long walk. This gives me hydration, calcium, and protein for muscle repair.
- *Stretch* – Do some gentle stretches, little and often, throughout the evening. Don't let your muscles seize up. 'Legs up the wall' is a favourite stretch of mine for the hamstrings and lower back, and it's also good for circulation and relieving cramps.
- *Move* – Keep moving at regular intervals throughout the evening to keep the muscles from shortening and to boost circulation to assist with muscle repair.
- *Elevation* – When sitting down for the evening – and especially once in bed – try to place a pillow under your feet to keep them elevated. You'll be thankful for this the next morning.
- *Bath* – A warm bath with Epsom bath salts will help to reduce the soreness and aches in your muscles. It will relax you and give your feet a well-deserved soak.
  (Remember: DON'T be tempted to rip the plasters off!)
- *Massage* – If you have no one to offer you a good back, neck, and shoulder rub, then do what you can yourself. Massage your feet and toes, thighs and

neck. A foam roller can be beneficial if you can tolerate it! This will increase blood flow to these tired muscles and assist with muscle repair.
I like to use a foot mask on my feet after a walk; this feels amazing and leaves them soft and moisturised.

- *Pain Relief* – When I've been hiking all day, I always take some paracetamol before bed as I know that the aches and pains can keep me awake.
- *Magnesium* – I like to use a magnesium spray on my calves and thighs post-hike. I'm not sure how much science there is behind this, but I think it makes a difference and enhances repair.
- *Gentle stroll* – Get outdoors the next day and take a gentle stroll. Keep the muscles moving; this will help with muscle repair and it will prevent the muscles from seizing up.

POST-HIKE STRETCHES

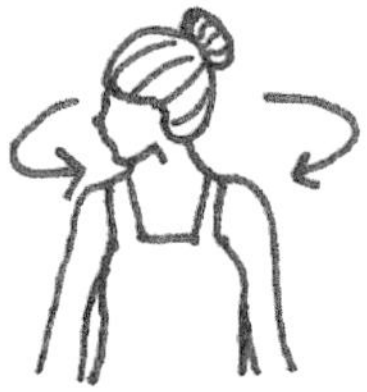

Neck Rotation

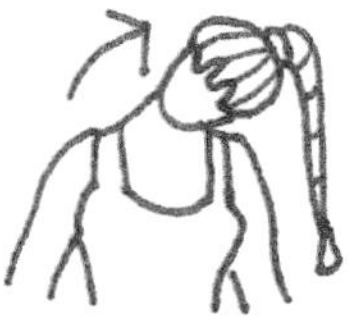

Neck Flexion

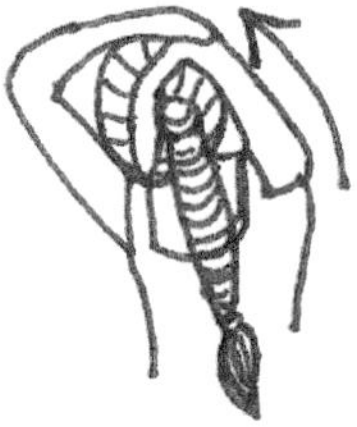

Lateral Stretch

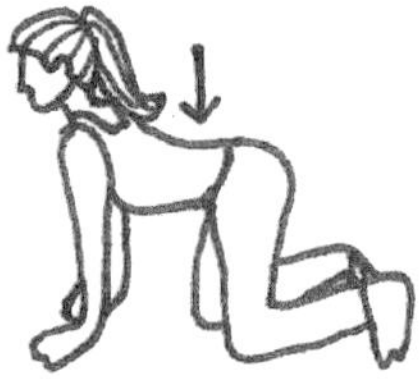

Cat Stretch

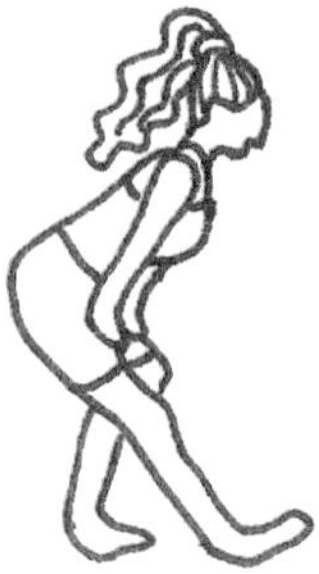

Hamstring

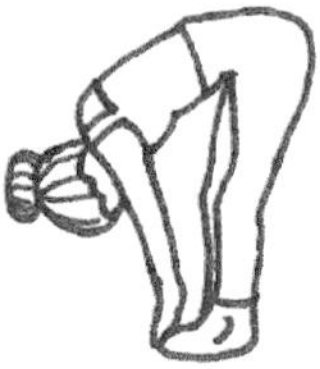

Spine Extension

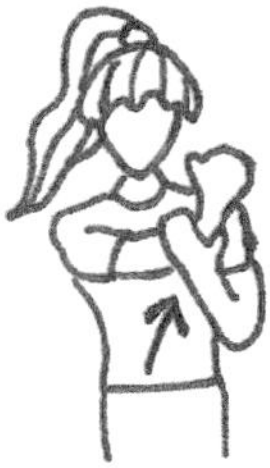

Triceps

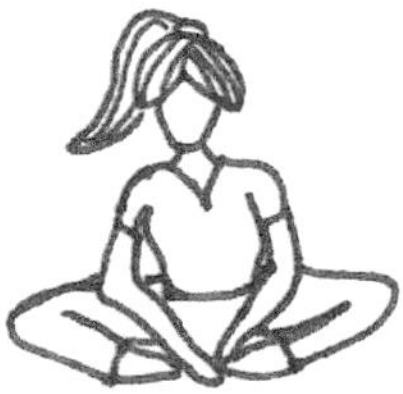

Inner Thigh

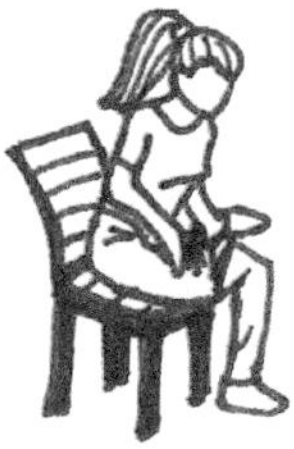

Hips

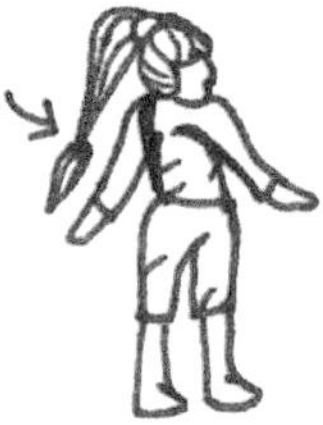

Thoracic

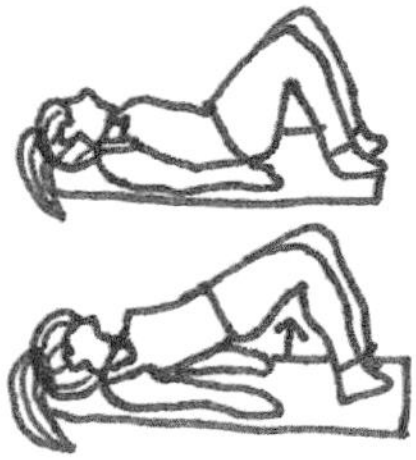

Bridges (lower back)

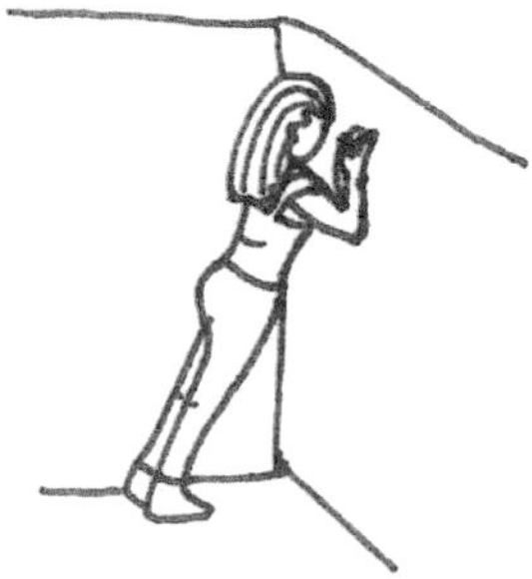

Calves

SAFETY

Your safety is paramount whether you're hiking alone or with others. Solo hiking does, of course, bring higher risks and vulnerabilities with it, but as long as you are sensible, know your limitations and don't hike where it is advised not to do so you should have no worries.

- Always tell someone where you're planning to walk and your estimated time of return. Then check in with that person when you're back so they can raise an alarm if they don't hear from you.
- Allow someone to track your phone so you can be found if you get into trouble or don't return.
- Ensure your phone is fully charged and that you have backup charging devices e.g. a battery bank or solar charger (and don't forget the leads!).
- Keep your whistle within reach in case you need to draw attention to yourself in an emergency.
- If you find yourself completely lost, try to retrace your steps (if possible) to where you went wrong. If that fails, use your compass to head in the general direction you're meant to be going and hopefully you'll come across something recognisable on your map to reorientate yourself.
- GPS apps or devices will be invaluable to you if you become lost, as it's not always easy to find your location when you've gone off-piste. (Always try to keep an eye on the paper map too, as technology cannot always be relied upon!)

- Identify places of safety on your route – e.g. pubs, farms, churches – where you can seek assistance and refuge if needed.
- Keep alert – If you need to wear earphones, try to just use them in one ear. You need to be aware and alert to your surroundings at all times.
- Check the map at regular intervals to confirm you actually are where you're supposed to be. It will be much easier to correct wrong turns if you know where and when you were last in the right place.

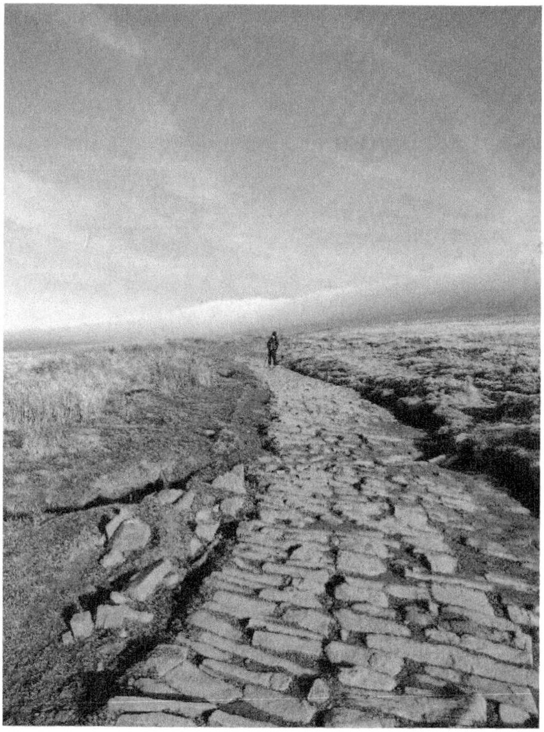

FELLOW HIKERS

Most people you'll meet on your hike will be doing it for the same reasons as you. They are there to enjoy nature and take some time out of the rat race.

- Some days you may not feel like chatting with everyone you meet, and that's fine. Just smile politely, bid them a good day, and be on your way. Other times it may be reassuring to see others and chat. Other hikers are often your best source of information and advice, if you need it, as well as assistance if you're lost or injured.
- Sometimes you'll come across a walker that may make you feel uneasy. Listen to your instincts and keep your distance. If possible, let them pass and keep them in front of you at all times; keep them in view but hang far enough back to not have to engage with them.
- Be bold and appear confident.
- If you feel threatened by another person out there, stay close to others or larger groups of people.
- Keep your phone and your whistle at hand.

Every person you meet is out there doing their own thing for their own personal reasons. You cannot know their situation. Try not to pre-judge, as you would not wish to be pre-judged yourself, and allow them the space to do what they're doing.

Tune into your own purpose, and use your instinctive nature to keep yourself safe.

DINING ALONE

This can be daunting for us women (and I'm sure some gents too), especially if it's not something you're used to doing.

However, if you're hiking alone there will be times when you need to visit a pub or café either for sustenance or for use of their facilities.

You may also be gasping for a cold beer on a hot day but might feel too self-conscious to go in alone.

I used to feel this way; I would just walk on past, wishing I was braver. Then either the hot weather and the calling for an ice-cold drink, or the cold weather and the need for some warm soup and shelter, got the better of me.

These days, I don't think twice about it, and I don't actually think anyone really notices or cares. With a rucksack at your side, it's obvious to others why you're there and it can even promote friendly conversation.

Firstly, I'd say cafes are easier than pubs – mainly because it's more common to see people drinking/eating alone in a café.

If you need to go to a pub for a meal, then maybe go earlier when it may be quieter, be sure to take a good book with you so you have something to distract yourself, and try to tuck yourself up in a little corner.

Test this out before your adventure. Challenge yourself and I promise you will feel empowered.

The other great bonus is that you get your own peace and quiet and you can sit and people-watch. You get to listen in to everyone else's conversation… usually making you quite glad that you're actually alone and that you have the courage and amazing ability to be so.

You'd be amazed at the number of people who will be in absolute awe of you!

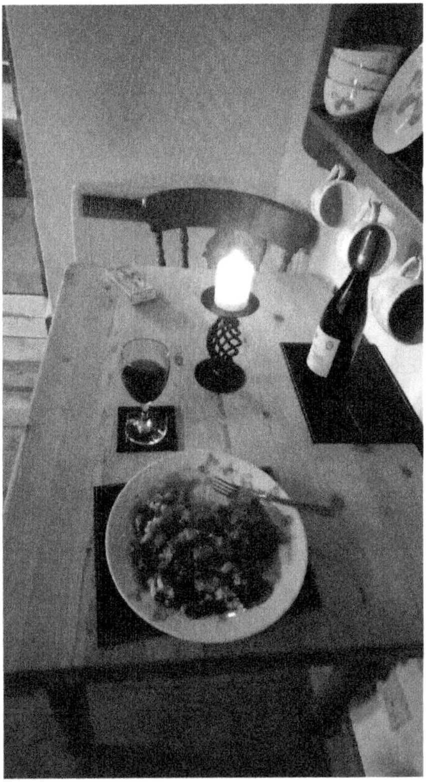

WHY DO WE WALK?

Humans evolved from quadrupedal to bipedal around five million years ago. There are many reasons and theories around why this evolution occurred, including the need for less energy when mobilising on two legs, the ability to reach higher into the trees, and freeing up our upper limbs and hands for using and crafting tools, as well as the development of fine motor skills for functional and social activity.

In more modern times we are obviously required to walk as a form of mobility, but it's also an activity we do for pleasure and fitness.

So, what is it that drives us humans to 'go out for a walk'?

- Studies show that regular walking in nature can change the structures within our brains. It increases blood flow to the brain, which releases neurotransmitters and endorphins that boost our mental health, alertness and mood. This can increase brain plasticity in memory and learning.
- A lack of movement and inactivity can cause physical concerns such as back pain, muscle wastage, joint stiffness, increased blood pressure, increased cholesterol, obesity, and mental fog. Moving your body in any way it allows you to will be of benefit.
- Walking offers a much lower risk of injury than running.

- Being outdoors can offer social connections with other humans and animals, whether in nature or in more urban settings.
- Our intake of vitamin D is increased by being out in the fresh air and sunshine.

Resilience is also an important factor, as planning and executing a walk builds strength. When you are wet, tired and hungry (and probably lost) and feel like giving up, what will you do?

There is no helicopter on standby that is going to drop you a line when you shout. You will have no choice but to continue until you get somewhere – and that place may be your destination, or it may be a place where you can call a cab or a friend, catch a train, or seek refuge. Give yourself the credit you deserve for pushing through and ask yourself: 'Do I still want to give up?' Tomorrow is another day, and part of your journey and your growth is pulling yourself out of those dark times.

This has been me on many occasions, but I always make a promise to myself that I will get to my destination and re-evaluate. Often, once you're dry, warm and fed, you can see more clearly and make a more rational decision.

Of course, there's nothing wrong with terminating your journey if your reasoning is right for you (especially if you have an injury that requires attention or rest).

As humans, we forget pain quickly (why else would women go on to have more than one baby??). Often, by the time you've reached your destination and the mist has cleared, you can congratulate yourself on your resilience and ability to push through and realise just what you went out there to do.

There's a whole host of studies and literature out there on this subject. It is a very interesting concept. For continued reading on this subject, check out the work of Shane O'Mara, Adam Bataineh, Francis Lecompte, and Annabel Streets.

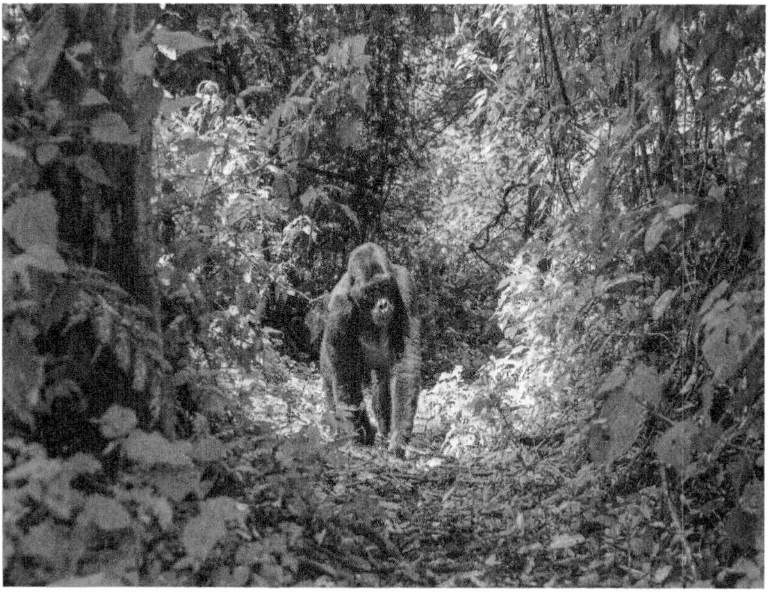

Hiking is so much more than just physical exercise. In fact, that is just a beneficial by-product for me. It is the quietness and space that I really thrive on, and the liberating feeling of achieving something I set out to do.

Walking makes me feel alive and soulful. I find myself identifying with all that is good in this life and the world we are living in. It helps me see that I have so much to be thankful and grateful for.

- Mindfulness – Being alone with nature is a fantastic way to get mindful. There are no daily distractions, no one demanding your attention, and nowhere else to be.
  You have set this time aside for yourself and there is no one to interrupt it (maybe put your phone on silent and only check it at intervals if you need to).
- Space – It gives you space to sort out all the junk and chatter in your head. You have hours to think and rethink things, and to process all the stuff that gets pushed aside in your busy everyday life.
- Be present – Take in the fresh air, the feel of it on your skin, in your lungs. Feel the sun on your face and the wind as it passes around you. Feel the energy of nature itself and draw your own energy from this.
- Being outdoors with nothing and no one but nature somehow fills me with hope.
  It turns the volume down on the sadness I may be feeling and the difficult challenges I may be

currently facing. It somehow lifts the mist so I can see some light and some hope, which totally fills my soul.

- Walking is sunshine for the soul and medicine for the mind.

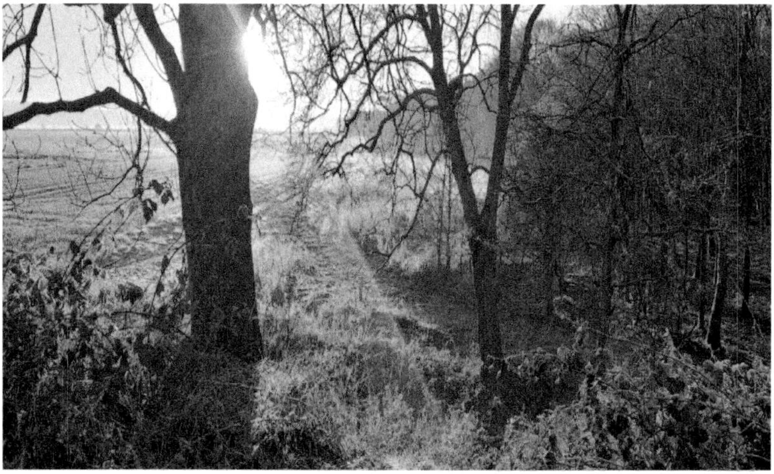

FOREST BATHING

What is forest bathing?

In the 1980s, the Japanese Ministry of Agriculture and Forestry created the term 'shinrin-yoku', which directly translates to "forest bathing" or "absorbing the forest atmosphere".

This new-age practice encourages people to simply spend time in – and be a part of – nature.

You can incorporate a slow, mindful walk in woodland and forested areas, where you are guided through a series of sensory experiences. This is proven to reduce stress and anxiety, which will calm your mind and body.

Often, walking into a forested area can be a contrast to other sections of your walk. Personally, I can feel a change as I move into the trees, as well as a sort of connection to their roots. It makes me feel grounded and in touch with the earth. It also makes me feel protected and gives me a sense of belonging with nature.

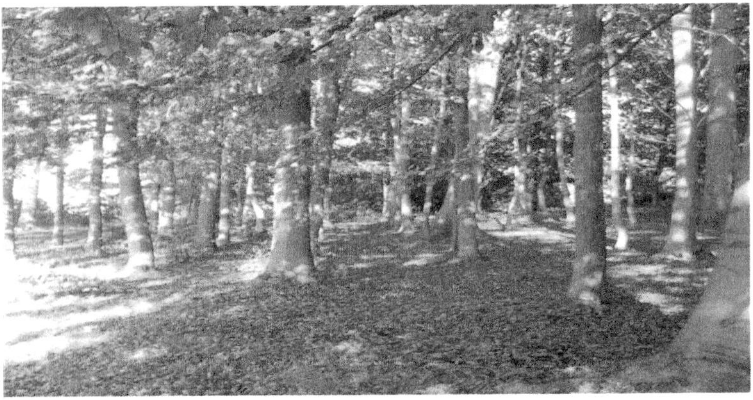

SMILE

When we're alone, and especially when we're feeling tired or fatigued, smiling is not at the forefront of our minds. However, if you make yourself smile (fake it until you make it, as they say), even if it's forced, there are so many benefits mentally and psychologically. It will even make you appear younger and apparently live longer.

Smiling not only offers an in-the-moment mood boost, but it also helps our bodies release cortisol and endorphins that provide numerous health benefits, including:

- Reduced blood pressure
- Increased endurance
- Reduced pain
- Reduced stress
- Strengthened immune system

All of the above are great benefits for hikers when it comes to our physical repair and well-being.

To smile at a stranger will automatically make them smile back (whether they want to or not).

Smiling activates tiny molecules in the brain that are designed to reduce stress. These molecules, called neuropeptides, facilitate communication between neurons in your brain. Also, when you smile, your brain releases dopamine, endorphins, and serotonin, which will promote positivity, make you feel good for the rest of the day, and help you sleep better.

You may even cause the one you smiled at to pass the smile forward... and then everyone's a winner.

Smile and the world will smile with you!

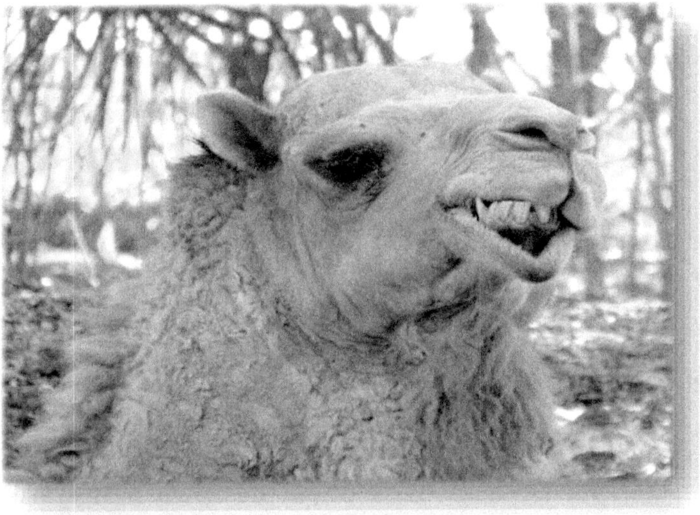

MY WALKING HEROES (a small selection)

Inspiration is all around us.

- The Brontës
  These talented young sisters walked for miles over their local moors to seek inspiration for their writing. They were not perturbed by the weather or the seasons, and I believe some of their most passionate literature was very much shaped by the environment in which they sought their inspiration.

- Dorothy Wordsworth
  This wonderful independent lady was well ahead of her time and she is a great inspiration to female solo walkers. She was an author, poet and diarist who influenced the course of English poetry. She had a passion for nature and the great outdoors, being a regular walker of great distances and challenging terrain. This no doubt had a direct influence on her works.

- Cheryl Strayed
  I will forever be in debt to this woman for documenting and recording her journey. Reading her book, *Wild*, was by far my biggest drive to leave my fears behind and get out there and walk. At the time of her book release, I was in a similar place in my own life and could relate to her and her experience on so many levels.

- Emma Rowena Gatewood (Grandma Gatewood)
  This incredible lady was the first woman to hike the entire Appalachian Trail (2168 miles)… in tennis shoes… aged 67! Legend. No more need be said.

- Raynor Winn
  If you haven't yet read her books then go get yourself a copy. A truly inspirational lady who found true solace in her walking adventures that were driven by homelessness and despair, and that changed her life – and her perception of it.

- Alfred Wainwright
  Alfred Wainwright (1907 – 1991) is best known for his *Pictorial Guide to the Lakeland Fells*, a seven-volume series describing the natural features, the routes of ascent and descent, and the views from the summits of 214 Lake District fells. He also plotted the much used and loved route across England from St Bees on the west coast to Robin Hood's Bay on the east coast, better known as the Coast to Coast Path.

  I am in possession of several of his books and have yet to execute many of his walks.
  He was reportedly a somewhat stubborn and particular man who liked things in order and on his own terms. I kind of like this about him.
  His wanderings in the fells were inevitably solo affairs as he supposedly couldn't stand most people.
  I am an admirer of his works and of his simplistic views.

MY WALKING INFLUENCES

There is no doubt in my mind that my dear mum has been the biggest influence on me in terms of walking – not being afraid of the weather and, well, just jolly well getting on with it!

When we were children, she would take us out regularly to walk in the woods or on the beaches. She would also ensure we had an annual holiday in the countryside, which would be mostly made up of countryside ambles and picnics. Indoors was only a place for sleep or a very rainy day!

In more recent years, we would go out walking together in the evenings and at weekends; living in the countryside offered countless opportunities for scenic walking. Having a collie dog always spurred us on too as they need plenty of exercise, and even after a long day's hike they are ready to go again. And, of course, they need to go out in all weather.

When my dear mum died in 2013, walking became my therapy. It was a space for me to grieve and relive my beautiful memories, and it helped me find some light during a very dark time.

Arthur Ransome – *Swallows and Amazons*

This book is one of the first childhood memories I have of the concept of adventuring beyond the back garden. It opened my eyes to how much fun could be had in the great outdoors and was definitely an influence on my love of adventure.

Enid Blyton – *The Faraway Tree*

The Faraway Tree was a regular bedtime read that opened my mind to where your imagination can take you… anywhere you like. I suppose this book has been a driver of my motto: If you don't go, you will never know!

Take the opportunities life gives you. They will always take you somewhere and enrich you.

Julia Bradbury

I just love watching this woman stomping all over the UK. Her walks have given me a great interest in parts of the UK I hadn't even thought of hiking and have been a huge inspiration for my adventures.

Simon Armitage – *Walking Home*

As I've mentioned elsewhere in this book, this chap inspired me to not only walk the Pennine Way, but to walk it in the wrong direction. For this, I am forever grateful.

Elizabeth Gilbert – *Eat, Pray, Love*

Some may say this is a cliché chick book (which has since been made into a film), but this book put a fire in me and opened my eyes to how much I am responsible for changing the things in my life that I'm unhappy with. It truly was a 'the world is your oyster' moment for me; it gave me the drive and direction to go it alone and take life by the short and curlies!

ENJOY

To gain the most from your experience, go out there with a positive and open mind. Know your limits and trust your instincts and you will have the most amazing of adventures and become the best, most enlightened, most liberated version of yourself.

- Use all of your senses:
- Smell the air, the mist and the earth.
- Listen to the wildlife – The birds, the bees, the sea (if you're on the beach), or the howling wind.
- Touch nature – Feel the leaves, the ground, the sand. Allow yourself to experience the amazing sensory feedback nature can offer you. Go hug that tree… yes, really! Give it a go.
- Taste – If the seasons are right (and if you're sure about what you're picking), taste the berries in the hedgerows, drink from the mountain streams (if you're high enough), and taste the salty air (if you're by the sea or lucky enough to stumble across some wild samphire or garlic).
- Look – Take in the beautiful scenery around you. Not through a camera or iPhone but through your own eyes. Soak it in and imprint it onto your memory. You can recall these moments when you're feeling stressed or angry or not coping with life.
- Open your mind and you can achieve anything you set out to do.
- "A walk in nature walks the soul back home" – Mary Davis.

- PENNINE WAY (PW)

The Pennine Way stretches for 268 miles (435 km) across some of England's bleakest northern uplands. It was the first official National Trail in England and is one of the UK's most famous long-distance walks.

I decided to hike the Pennine Way in May/June 2015. My inspiration and motivation for this was reading Cheryl Strayed's book, *Wild*. Having recently lost my mother to cancer, her story resonated with me and I was truly struck.

Before this, going on a lone venture in this way was only ever a dream to me and something only other (brave) people did. Her story made me believe it was something any of us can achieve – if we allow ourselves the chance to believe we can.

Living in England, I obviously didn't have the wildlife threats Cheryl encountered, so my journey was a tamer version. Nevertheless, it gave me a goal, and just the planning alone excited me.

I was very organised. As it wasn't something I'd ever experienced before, in order for me to succeed I felt like I needed to be prepared for every eventuality.

I used the A-Z Pennine Way map book, plus websites and blogs on the internet, to plan my route.

I decided to do this from north to south. This unusual idea of hiking the PW (as it's mostly done south to north due to the weather/winds) was given to me by an English poet, Simon Armitage. In 2012 he released a book called *Walking Home*, where he walked the PW from north to south, taking him back to his homelands.

This made sense to me, to be walking towards home rather than away from it.

My most memorable section of this trip was day three from Bellingham. Being day three, my feet and body were still in shock as to what I was asking them to do. My feet were covered in blisters, I ached all over, it had been pouring with rain so all my kit was damp, my boots were wet on the inside, I had burnt a hole in my tent door with my stove, and I was feeling mighty miserable.

On leaving the campsite that morning, still in the pouring rain, I dropped my map in a puddle and – not long after – was chased through a field by a herd of cows. In fear for my life, I had to jump a fence into a ditch and was promptly covered in mud and nettle stings. Needless to say, I was not happy. I actually sat down and wept! For all these reasons, this stands out as probably the worst moment of this whole adventure.

When I eventually pulled myself together and was looking for an alternative footpath, the farmer came along. I thought he was going to give me a telling-off for being off-track and on his land but, instead, he whistled for his dogs to jump down from the back of his quad bike and signalled for me to jump on. I wasn't going to refuse this, so he escorted me through his cattle to the other end of the field. Although I was unimpressed with him stopping in the middle of the herd to explain how dangerous cows can be, I was eternally grateful for his kindness.

I found shelter in a barn in a farmyard a little further along the trail, and on arrival I found a sofa, a toilet (even a shower!), a kettle with sachets of hot chocolate and soup, some handmake cakes, and a sign saying: 'Welcome, stay as long as you need.' At this point, I wept again! Although for different reasons. I was so totally humbled by the warmth, affection, and thoughtfulness of others. While I was there I had a little word with myself, and found the strength to shake myself off and continue.

This bittersweet day will always be at the forefront of my memories of that trip, as well as being a constant reminder of my inner strength whenever I need to dig deep. It also reminds me how powerful the kindness and compassion of other people can be.

Some tips I would suggest for planning a multi-day hike:

- Know your route and identify a realistic daily mileage, bearing in mind the location of the accommodation.
- Book your accommodation if possible and let them know your contact and approx. ETA to avoid panic and disappointment.
- This isn't essential, but I wasn't sure what I would find in the way of shops/supplies en route (though in actual fact, there were plenty), so I sent forward

packages to myself at intermittent campsites containing dried foods, plasters, etc.

- After two or three days I realised I'd packed too much that I just wasn't going to need. Therefore, I sent a package back home with clothes and items that were weighing me down.
- Underestimate rather than overestimate your daily mileage. When you're walking for consecutive days you need to allow some rest periods, and walking from dawn till dark day after day can become tiring and relentless. Having an easy day is a well-earned luxury.
- On short days (10 miles or less) I would carry my pack, but on the longer days, I arranged for it to be carried on to my prospective campsite with the Sherpa Van.

  I cannot recommend this enough; it made those long days far more enjoyable.
- My sister joined me for three days midway. This gave me the push I needed, and spurred me on to get to where I was meeting her in those early days when I was still adjusting, had broken feet, and felt like giving up. If possible, have a friend or loved one waiting for you at the end. This is such a driver to keep going, and sharing the finish line with someone is priceless.
- I would suggest doing a mini trip as a test run if possible. I took three days and planned my average mileage coverage per day. This was an invaluable eye-opener for me in terms of what I actually needed to pack, my footcare, and my realistic daily

distance. I totally overestimated what I could do, as well as the weight of my pack, and actually broke myself. From this I learnt many lessons – both practical and personal – and without it I may not have succeeded in my venture.

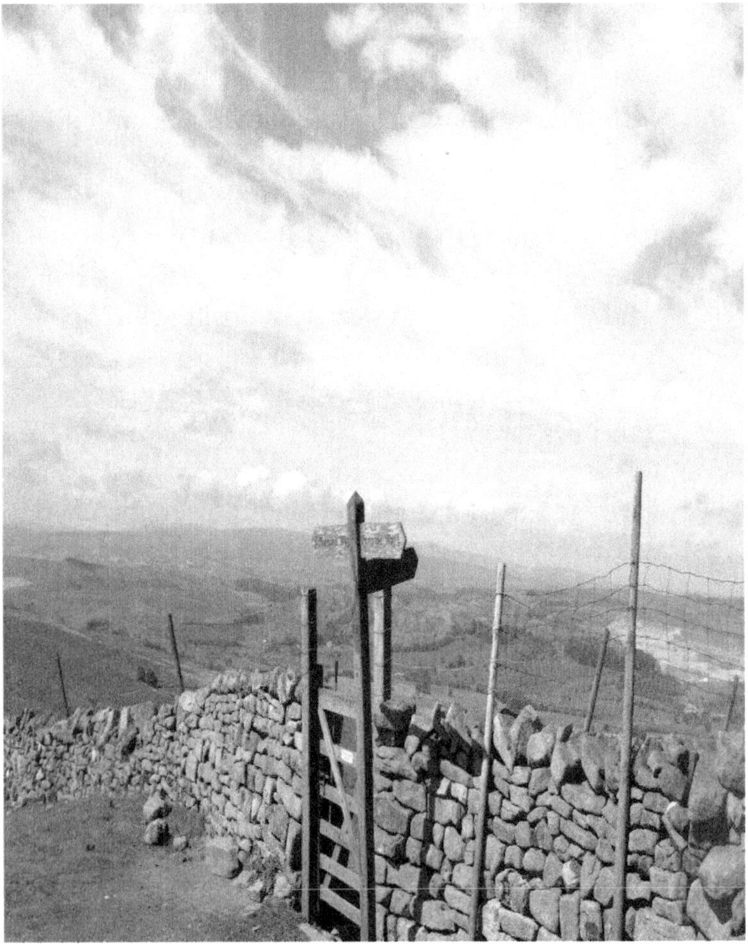

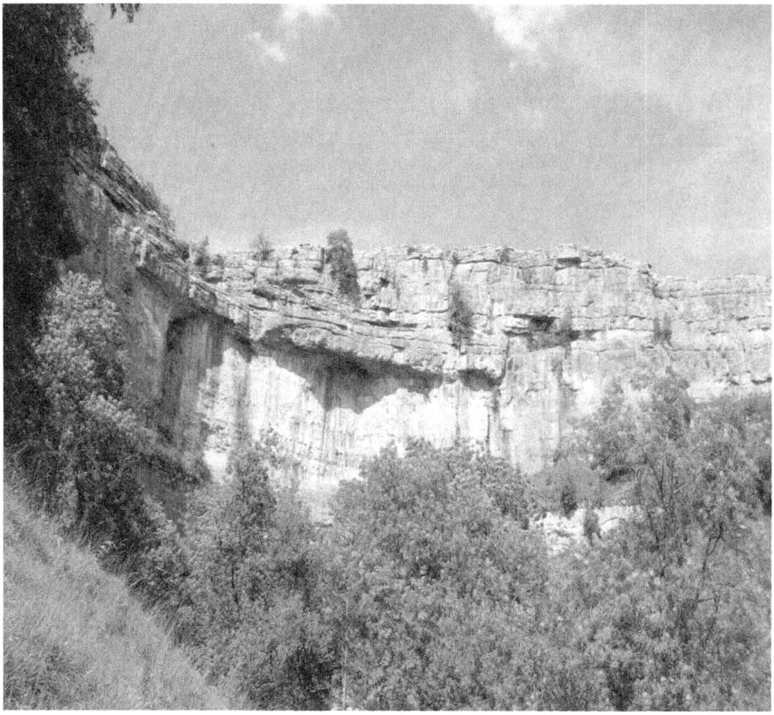

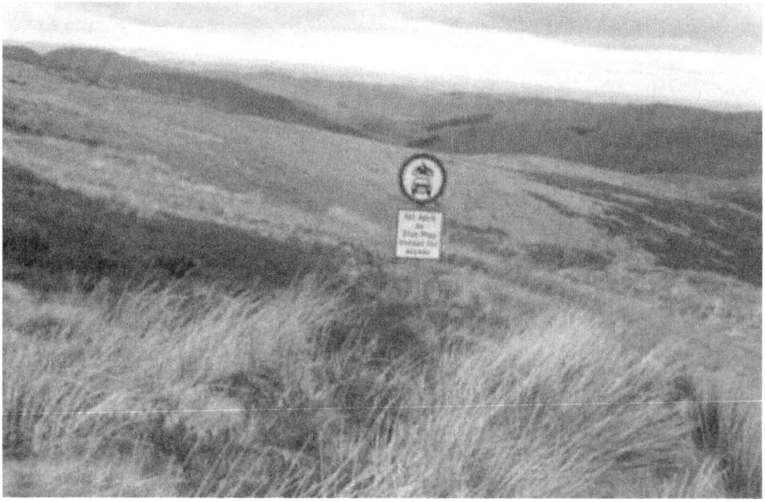

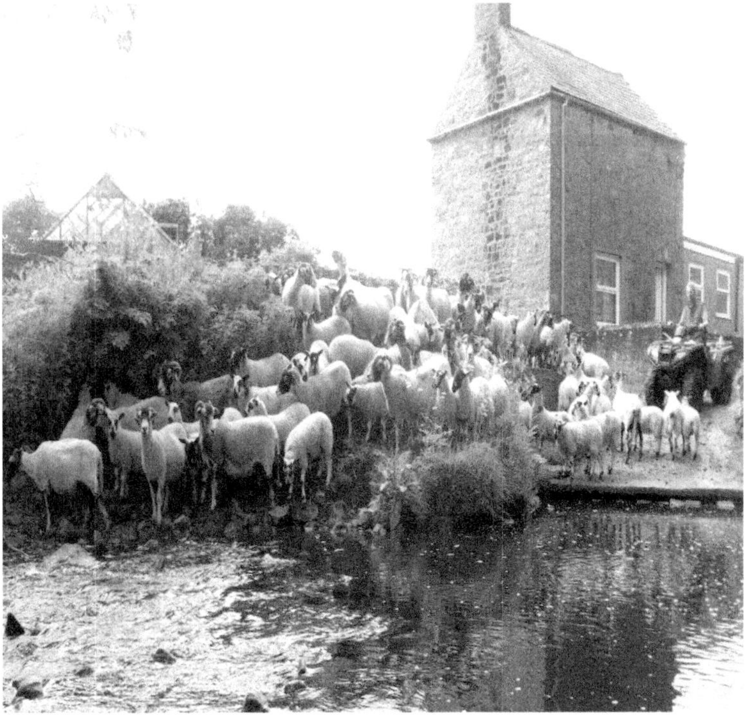

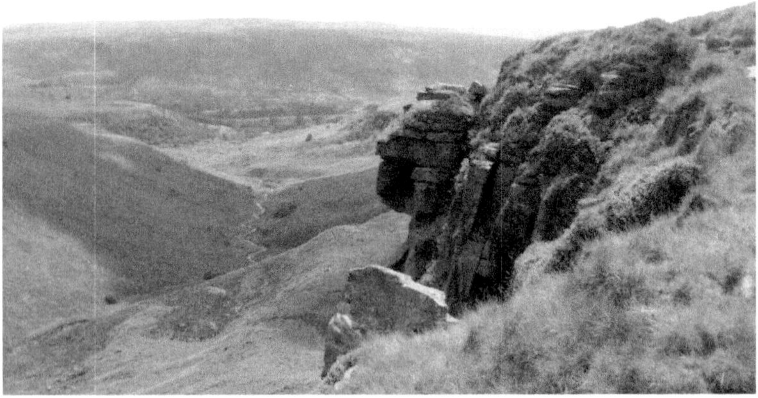

- COAST TO COAST (C2C)

England's Coast to Coast footpath is a 192-mile trail made up of dozens of existing footpaths, bridleways, minor roads, and other rights of way crossing the breadth of England, from St Bees in Cumbria to Robin Hood's Bay in North Yorkshire.

This stretches over the Lake District in the west, through the Yorkshire Dales, and across to the North York Moors and to the east coast. It offers a variety of terrain including mountains – Kidsty Pike (780m) being the highest, unless you're crazy enough to tag on Helvellyn (950m), descending via Striding Edge to day three… as we naively did! – beautiful lakes, valleys, and moorlands.

I hiked this in June 2021. It has since been recognised as an official British National Trail.

Whilst hiking the PW, I came across an intersection with the C2C at Keld, where I met other travellers walking in the other direction. This was my first real encounter with this path and I was intrigued.

After completing the Pennine Way in a vertical direction, I thought it would be good to traverse the country the other way (horizontally). So began my research into this newfound National Trail.

The idea of starting on the west coast of the country and finishing on the east (and carrying a pebble from one sea to the other, if you follow the tradition) captured my imagination. I planned my journey in much the same way as the PW, however, for this trip I decided to treat myself to B&Bs /hostels instead of camping. I have to say, I found this much more enjoyable and comfortable, but obviously it was a more expensive way to travel.

As I had less luggage than when I was camping, I decided to carry my gear with me along the route... this was, until my sister (who joined me for the first five days) offered to take my pack onto the next B&B when she left for home one morning. It was then that I realised how much freer and more comfortable this was, so I treated myself to the Packhorse Baggage transfer service. Some may call this cheating... I would say, 'If you can, then why not??'

My memories of this adventure were far more pleasant than the PW. I think having had such good weather (only half a day of rain) made all the difference to my daily walking, and I didn't really experience a 'bad' day. Of course, arriving each evening somewhere warm and dry, with a hot shower/bath, a hot meal, a space for me to dry my kit and an amazing sleep in a soft warm bed made this a much more enjoyable experience. My evenings were relaxing and therefore my recovery from each day was much better.

I was also well trained this time, having learnt from previous experiences and knowing what to expect.

Much like the PW, I found that to have someone meet you midway and then at the end is an amazing incentive to keep going. It was often the thought of seeing these beautiful familiar faces that got me through the tough days.

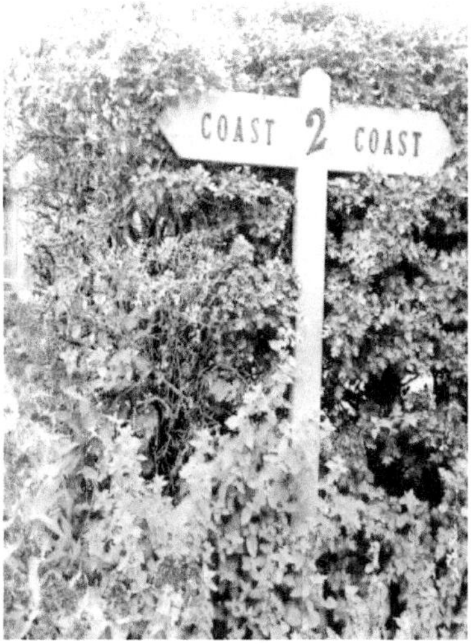
COAST 2 COAST

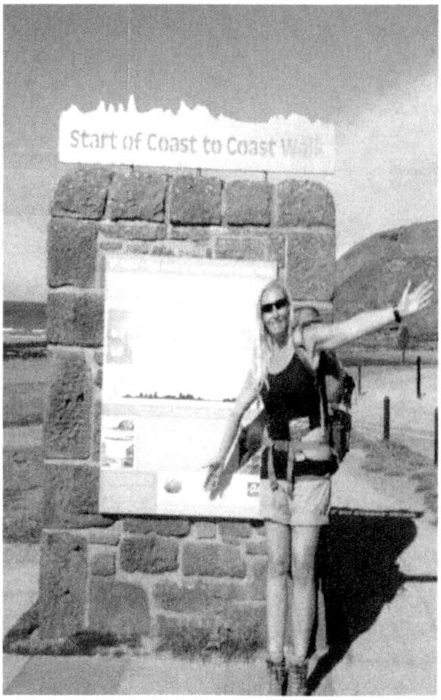
Start of Coast to Coast

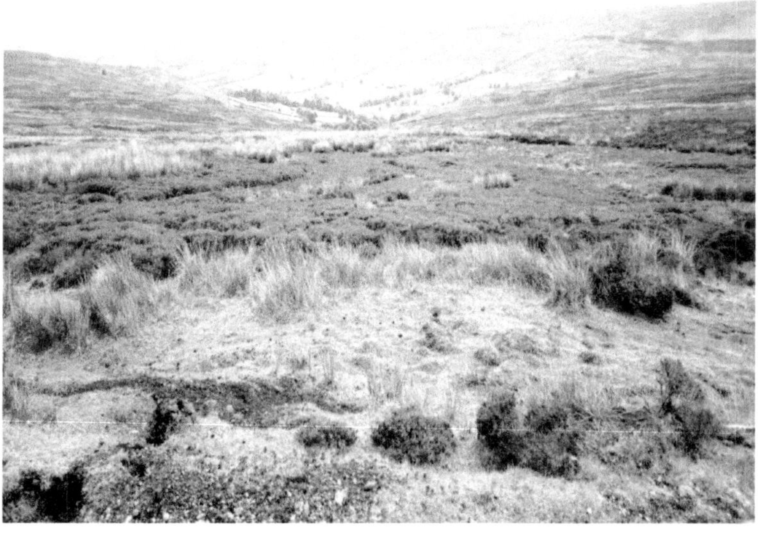

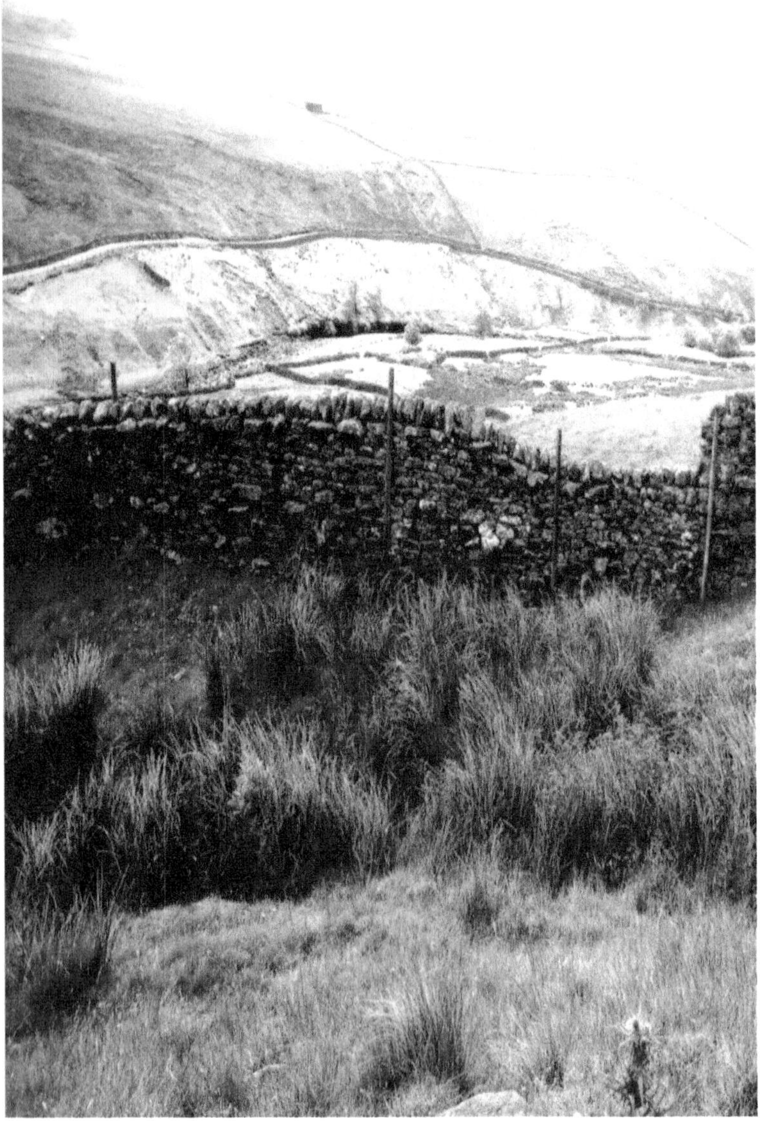

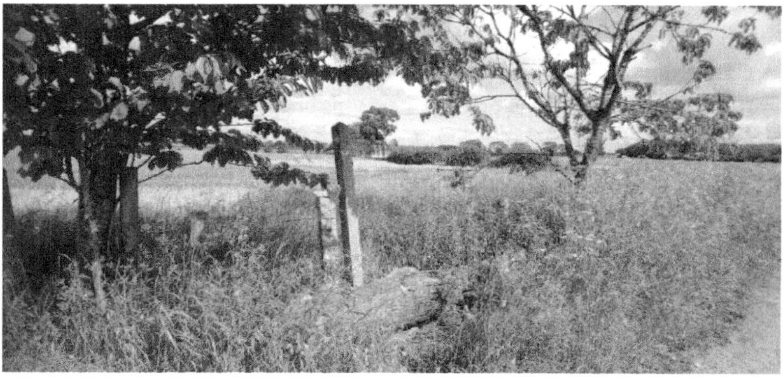

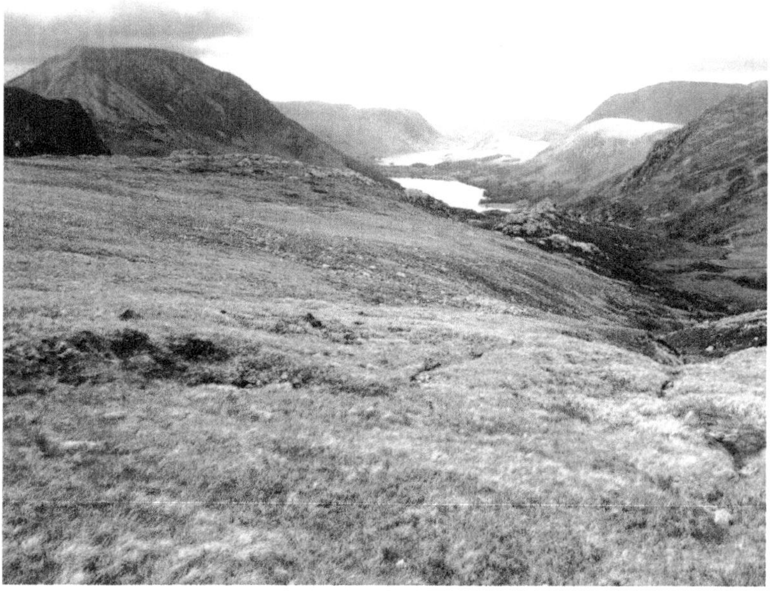

- PEDDARS WAY

The Peddars Way starts in Suffolk at Knettishall Heath Country Park and follows the route of a Roman road for 48 miles (79 km) to Holme-next-the-Sea on the North Norfolk coast, meeting the Norfolk Coast Path.

This was a three-day hike for me (two nights), and this time I carried all my gear and camped. This was the reason for reducing my daily mileage, which made it a more enjoyable experience.

The weather, again, was kind. I hardly saw a soul the entire trip (until I got to the Norfolk coastline, that is).

There were some very remote areas – such as the plantations through Thetford Forest – that were not the most inspiring... However, there were plenty of beautiful sights and wildlife to see along the way. If you're considering doing this, just be prepared for solitude.

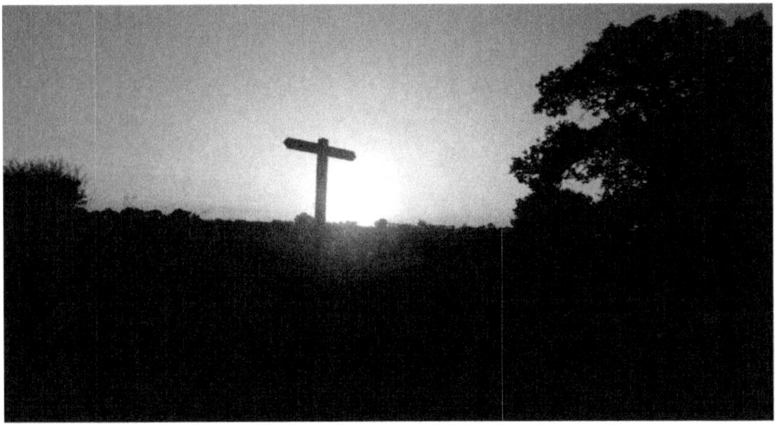

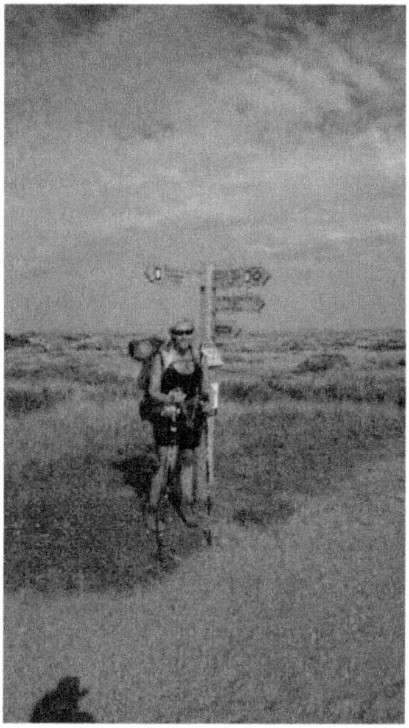
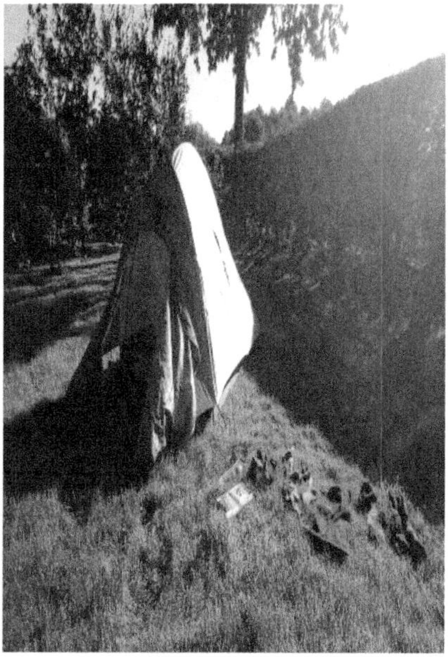

- NORTH NORFOLK COASTAL PATH

The Norfolk Coast Path is 84 miles (135 km) of walking from Hunstanton to Hopton-on-Sea through fantastic scenery and landscapes. The majority of the trail runs through the Norfolk Coast Area of Outstanding Natural Beauty (AONB).

Being a Norfolk lass, I have spent many a time out here walking this path. It is absolutely stunning and wild in many of the remote sections, with miles of stretching sands where there is rarely a soul to be found.

The later section, from Cromer to Hopton, has only recently been added and has few reviews or literature. This section is much less known and, I have to say, much less accommodating. There is very little in the way of accommodation along the route, and most of the route is along sand or sand dunes.

Seaside towns such as Cromer, Hunstanton, and Great Yarmouth are busy – as to be expected – but they're great places to find an assortment of food, pubs, and entertainment, if that's what you're seeking.

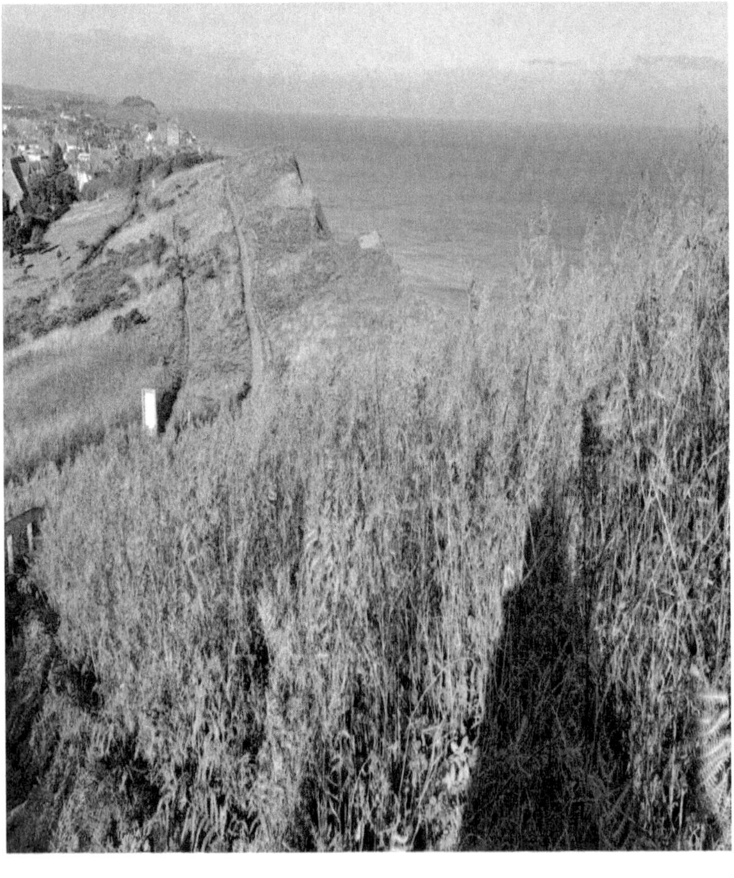

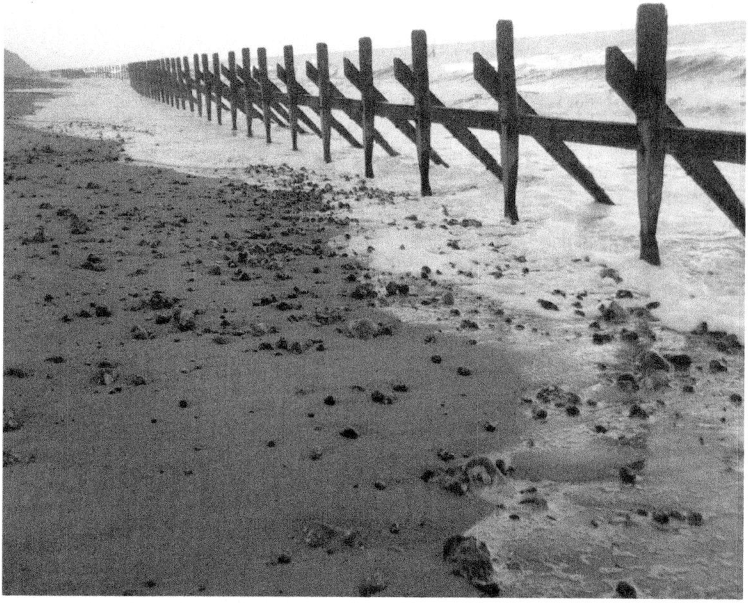

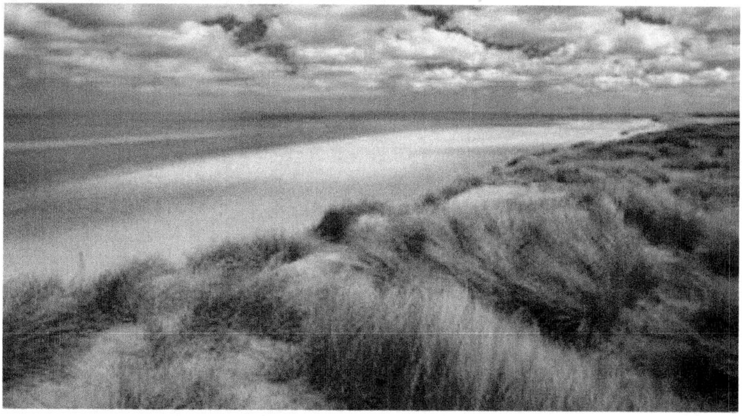

- DERBYSHIRE PEAKS WALKING

If I have a free weekend and am in need of a good stomp then I can often be found out in the Derbyshire Peaks. Living in Norfolk is beautiful, but it is quite flat. When I get my mountain itch and need to feel the energy of the hills, this is my nearest outlet.

The three highest peaks in Derbyshire are Black Hill, Bleaklow and Kinder Scout. That said, there are 322 peaks in total to choose from, with a variety of terrain from the dark peaty peaks (and bogs) to the white gentler slopes and the moorlands.

Being here, I feel home; it's a place I visited often as a child and I can never ever get bored of it. There are endless options for walking and camping along with hostels, B&Bs, and holiday cottages. These days, some areas are particularly busy with tourists so I try to keep away from them at peak times. I always feel safe when in these lands and it will always be my go-to escape.

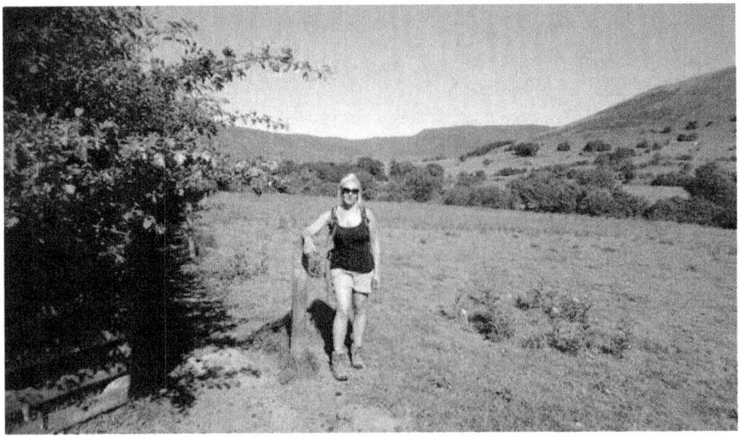

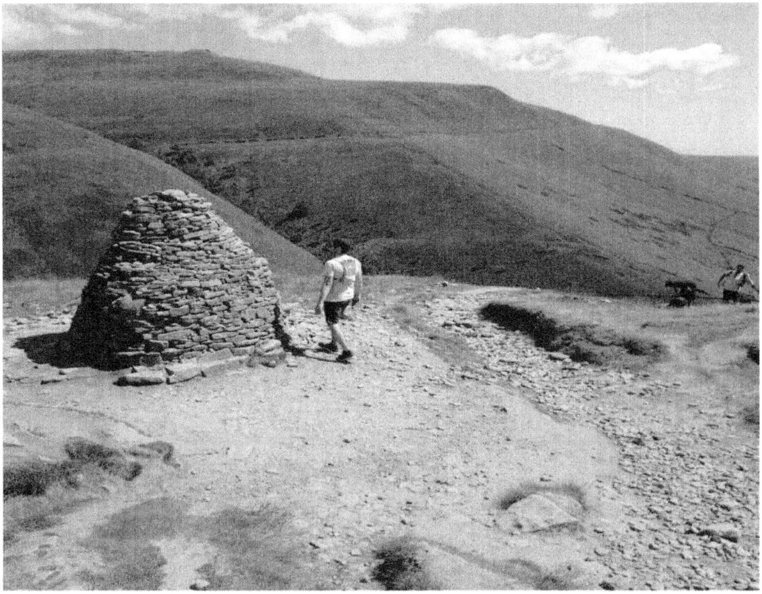

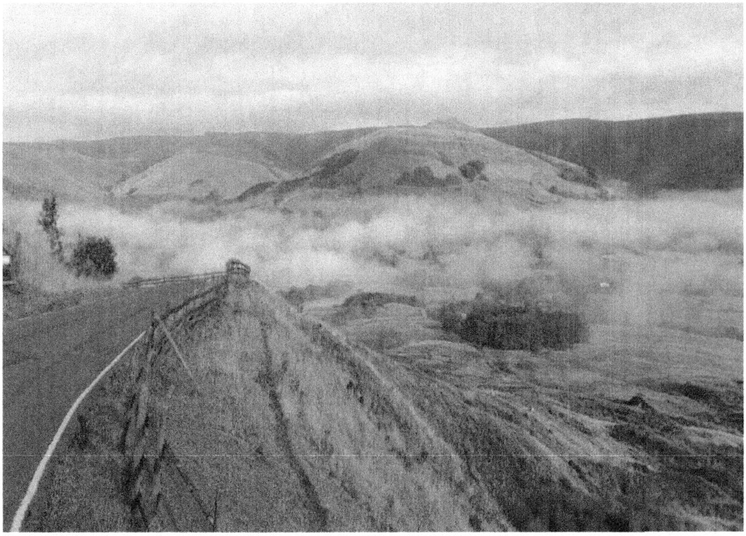

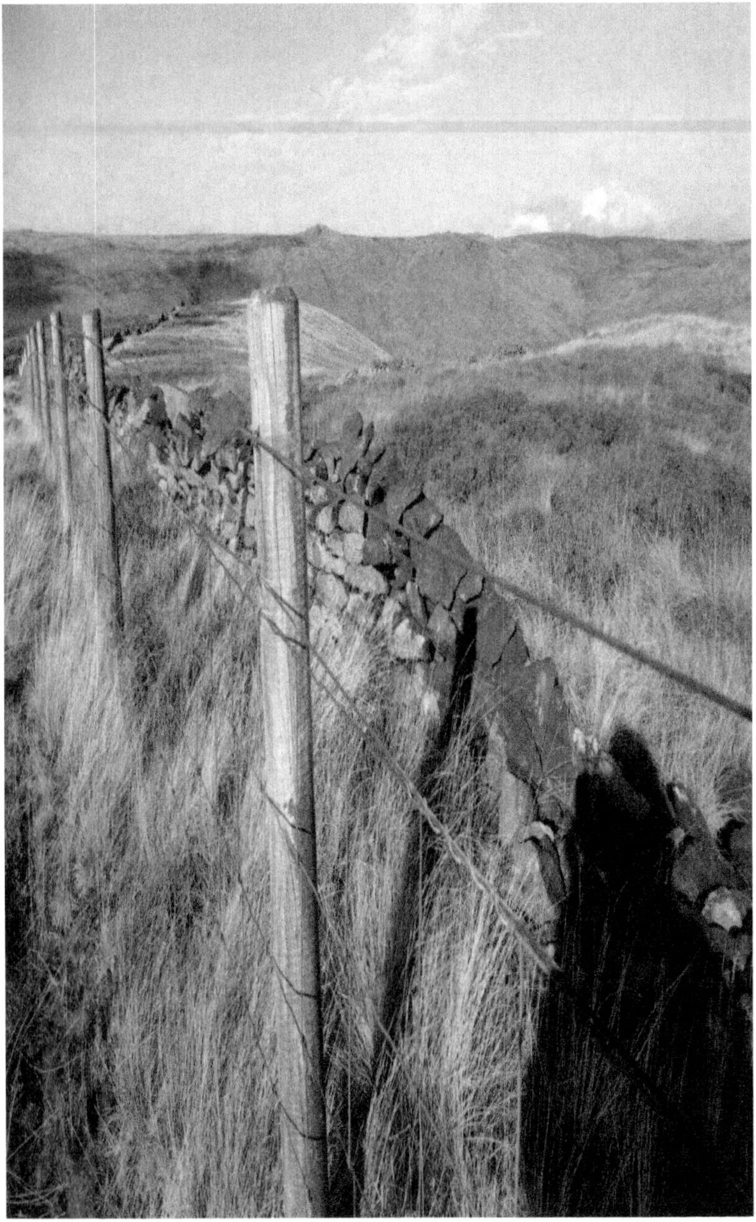

- YORKSHIRE THREE PEAKS

The mountains of Whernside (736m), Ingleborough (723m) and Pen-y-ghent (694m) are collectively known as the Yorkshire Three Peaks. The circuit trail is approx. 24 miles in total, and the famous Three Peaks Challenge is to complete the circuit in under 12 hours.

The first time I did this was in 2009, when it was not so well marked. We got lost in a bog for some time and took a while to get ourselves back on the path. This was on a scorching hot day, with not enough sunscreen or water, and I think we took around 13 hours to complete it. There was a lot to be learnt from this!

Since then I have completed the challenge five or six more times – once in thick snow, when I only saw a handful of people all day. It is so well signposted now that it's nearly impossible to get lost... even for me!

I've started the route in various places in order to mix it up. I have yet to do it in reverse, however, as I'm put off by the idea of a sea of people constantly walking at you.

I would suggest trying one or two of the peaks first to see if it's your thing. Also, if you're able, go mid-week as the weekends are like Piccadilly Circus.

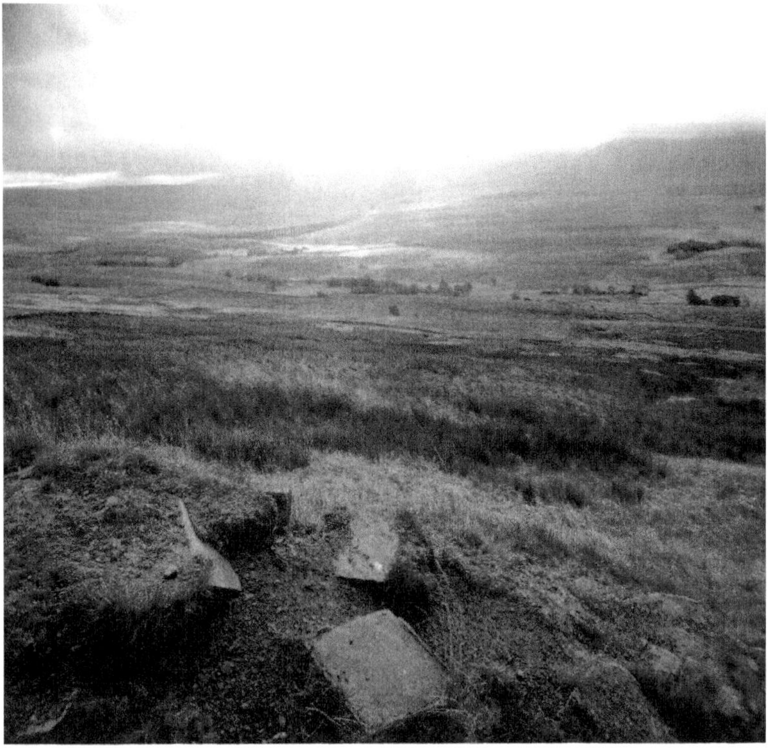

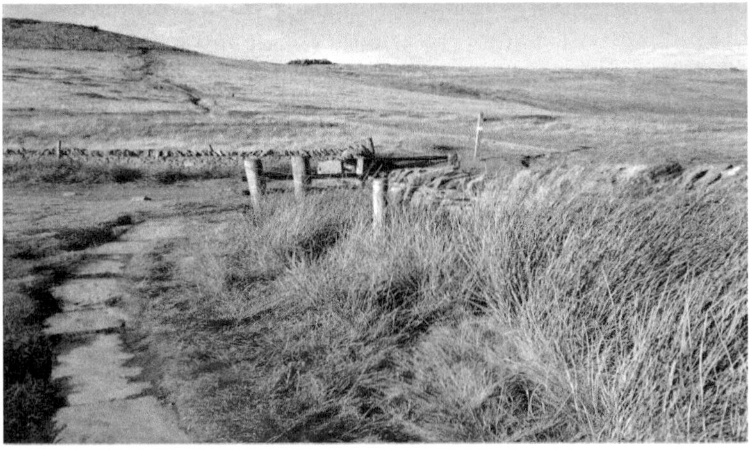

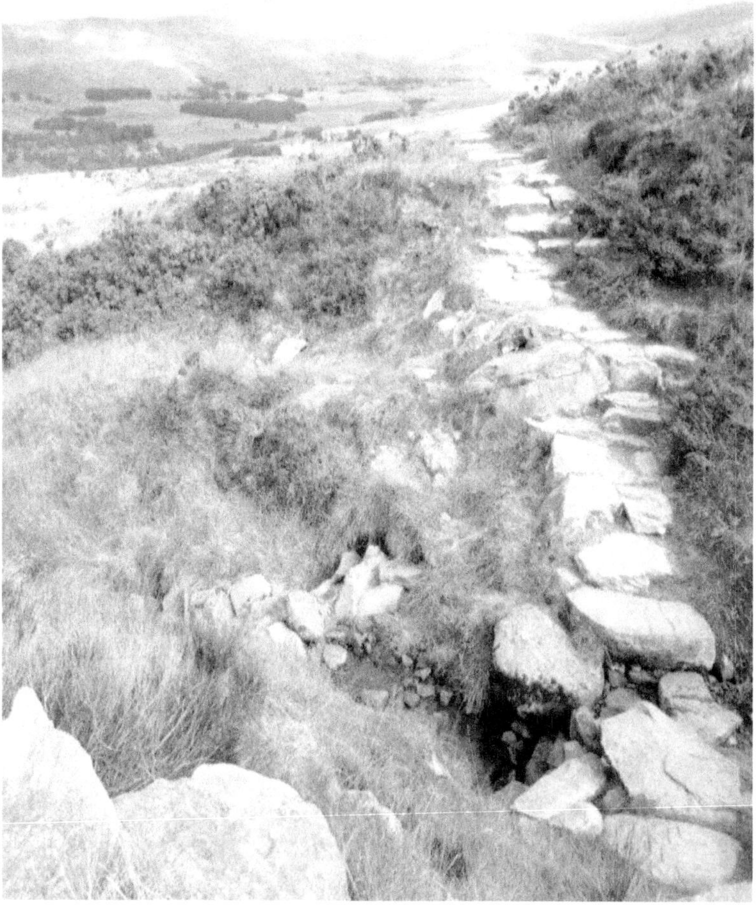

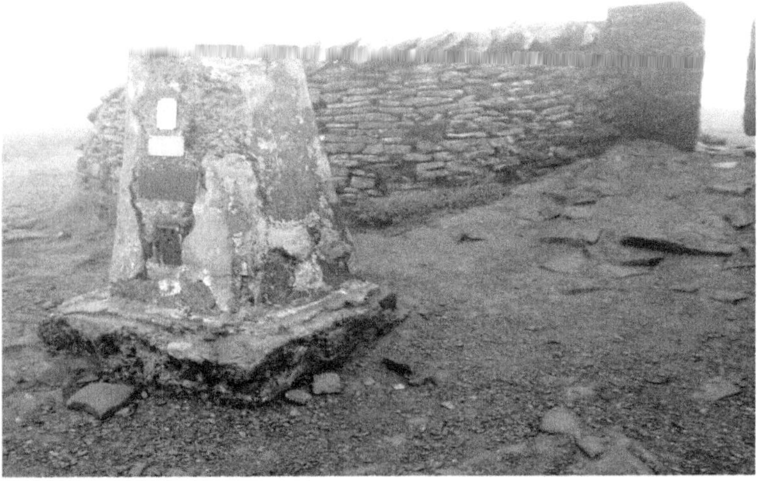

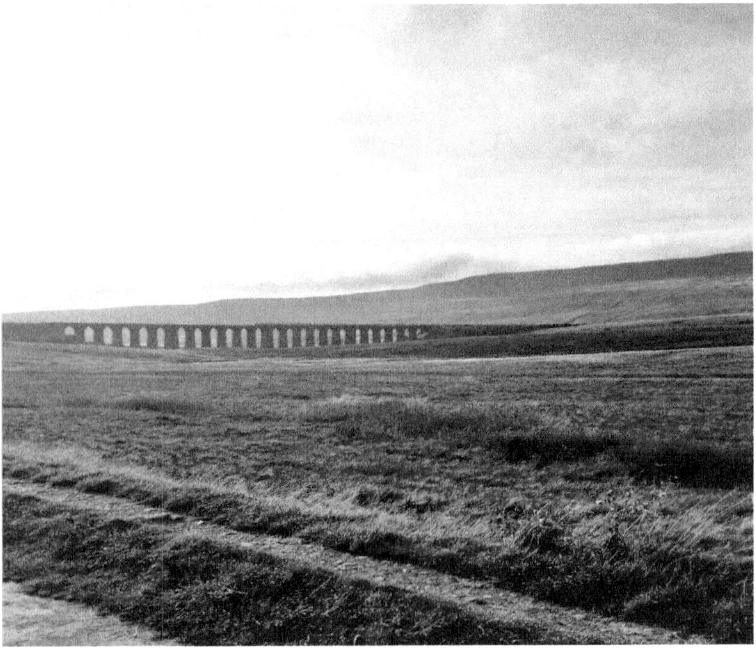

- NATIONAL THREE PEAKS (SCAFELL PIKE, SNOWDON, BEN NEVIS)

The three mountains that make up the National Peaks are the highest in England, Scotland and Wales: Snowdon, in Wales (1085m); Scafell Pike, in England (978m); and Ben Nevis, in Scotland (1345m), totalling 23 miles in three stages, a total ascent of 3064m.

I have only ever done these as individual hikes and not as the challenge suggests (within 24 hours).

Last time I did Scafell Pike we got somewhat lost and found ourselves out there in the darkness. That was an interesting experience...

There are a variety of ways to summit this mountain. It is fairly well pathed on the major routes, but it's worth checking your map and compass to ensure you descend the way you intend to.

I first did Snowdon when I was about 14 years old, in very pathetic slip-on velvet shoes! They were fashionable at the time... What can I say!

This, again, has a variety of routes. The main route runs alongside the mountain railway and is very clearly marked.

Ben Nevis I have only done once. This is the highest of the three, and the path runs up the mountain in a zigzag fashion. It is a fairly easy walk and the best bit is the pub at the bottom.

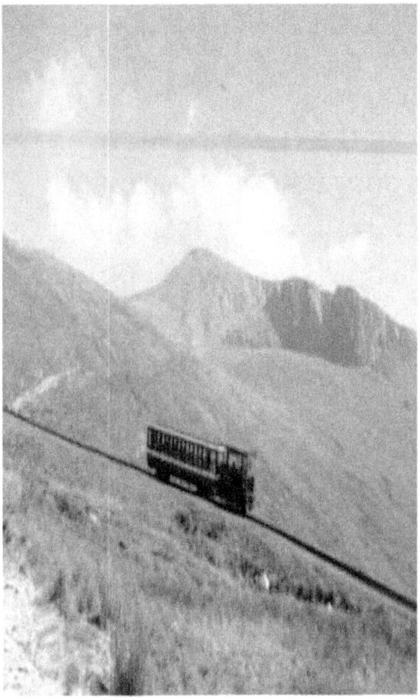

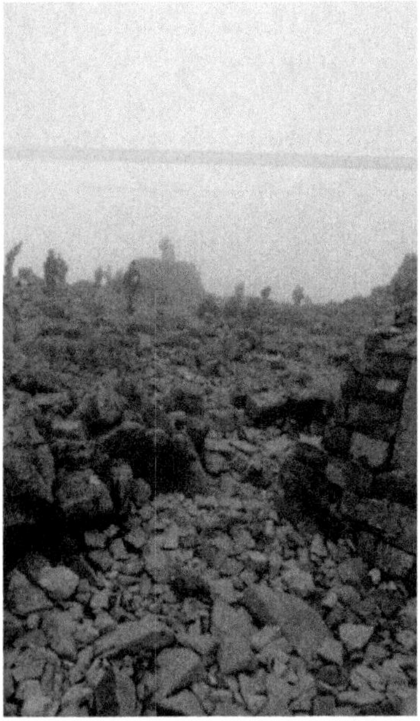

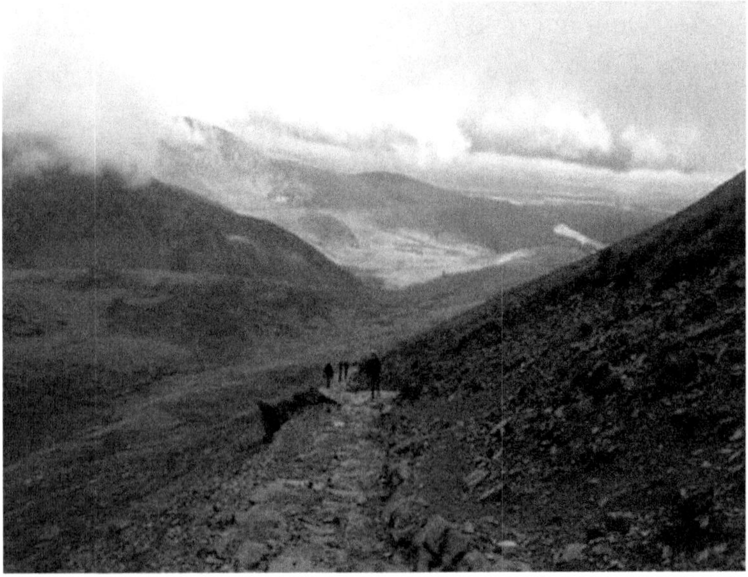

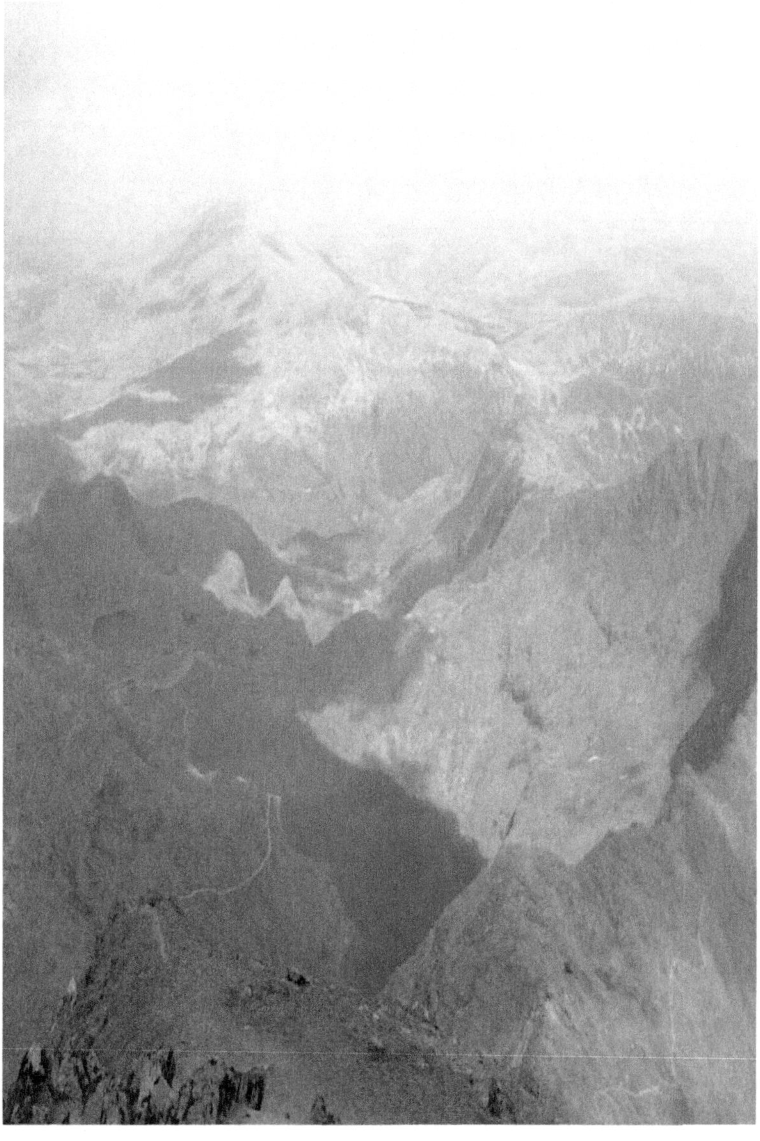

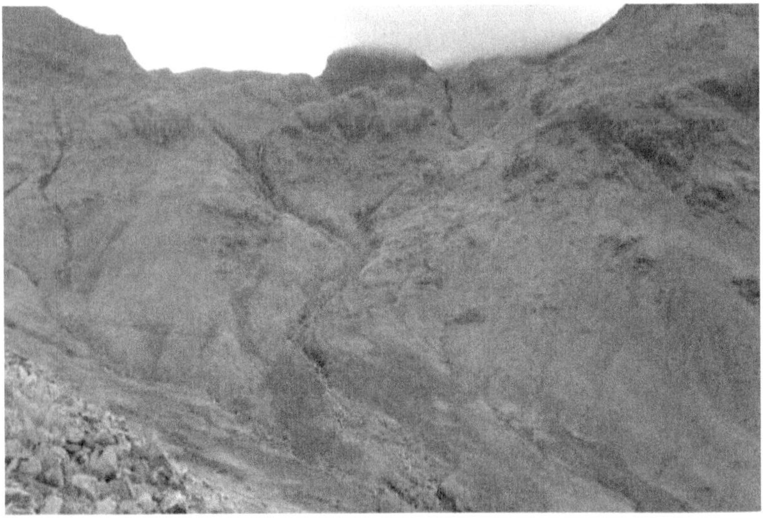

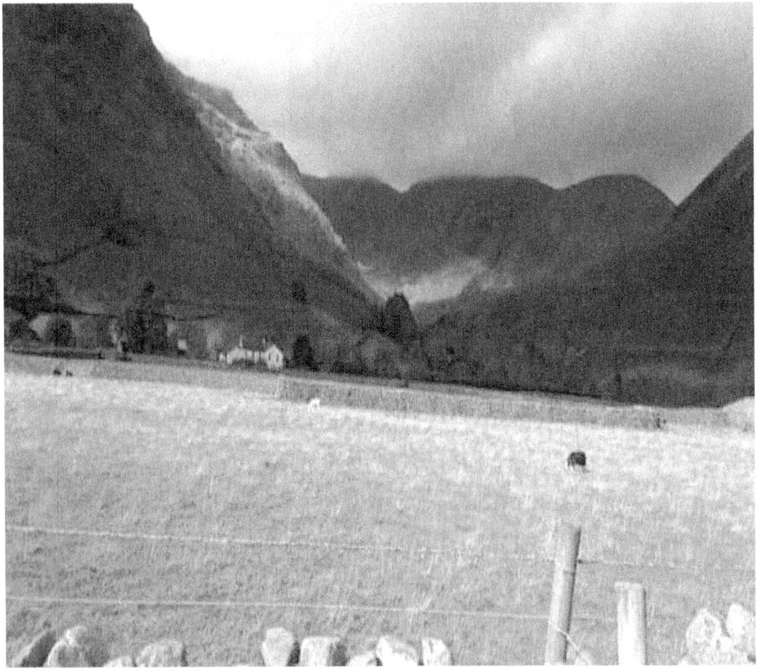

- PEN Y FAN (BRECON BEACONS)

This is the tallest mountain in South Wales (886m). There are many routes up it, but the main route from the Storey Arms is by far the most popular and well-laid path. It lies within the Brecon Beacons so is surrounded by beautiful mountain ranges.

This is a good one to start with; given that it begins at 440m above sea level and is approx. a 4-mile round circuit, it's not too long. There are wild ponies on the route and, although the pub is no longer a pub, there is often a coffee/burger bar at the bottom.

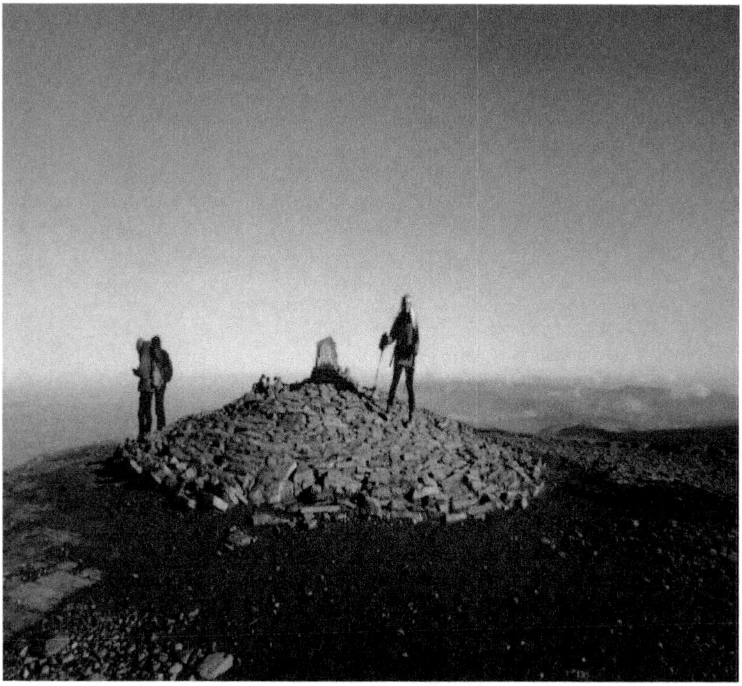

- NORFOLK WALKS (LOCAL)

Being a Norfolk girl, I have stomped pretty much all over this county. We are so very lucky here to have the coastline and the Norfolk Broads along with lots of rural areas and countryside.

There are thousands of pubs to plan your walks around and, of course, thousands of churches, which are always places of interest or places of respite if nothing else.

There are many trails and marked footpaths to execute, offering over 1200 miles of walkways. To name a few of my favourites: The Norfolk Mountain (National Trust), The Weavers' Way, The Marriott's Way, The Paston Way, The Boudicca Way, The Norfolk Coastal Path... and the list goes on.

They say Norfolk is flat... don't be fooled...

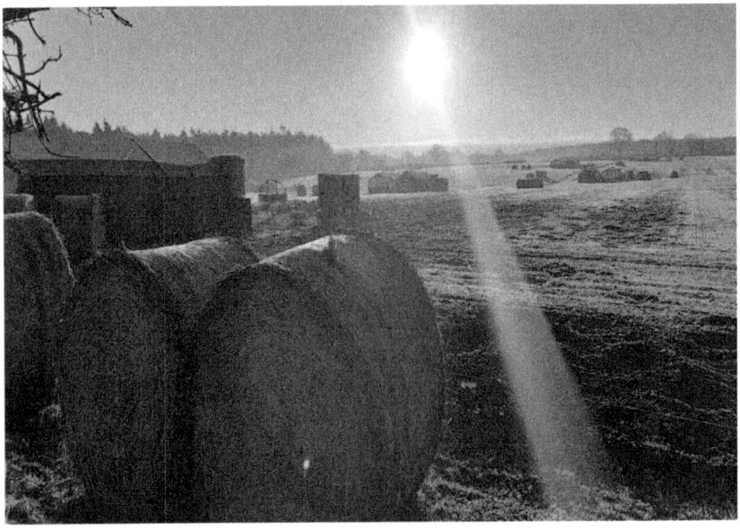

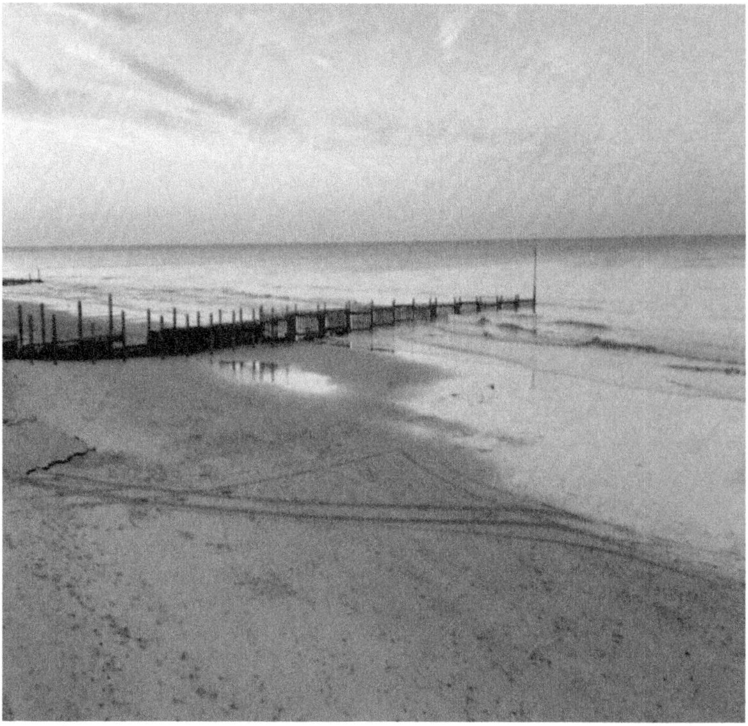

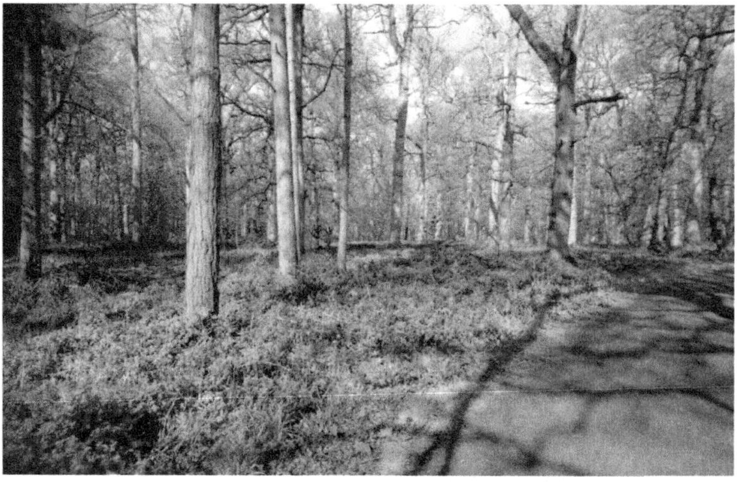

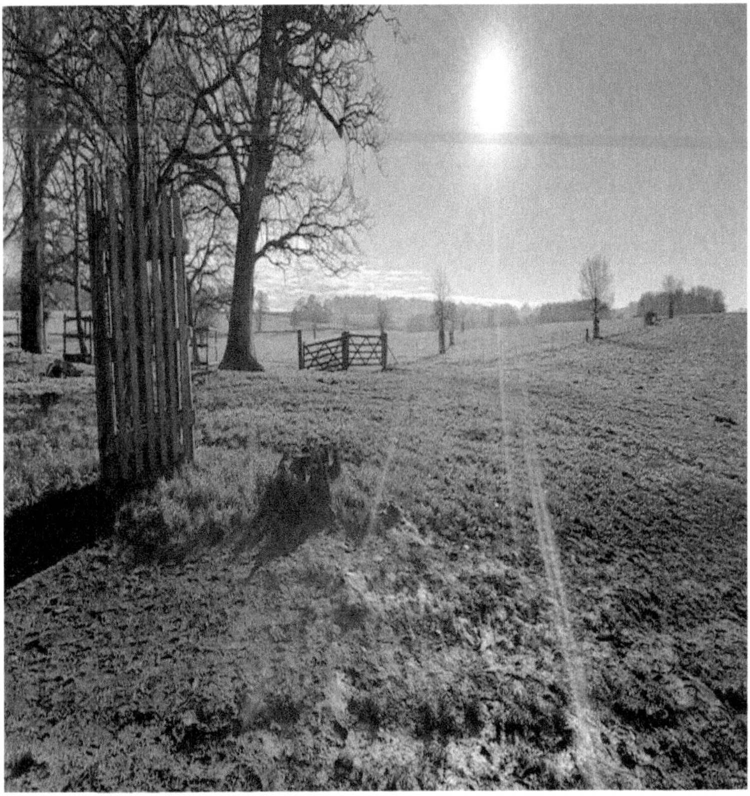

- LINCOLNSHIRE WOLDS WAY

The Lincolnshire Wolds – which can be described as an elevated area of open countryside – are possibly one of Lincolnshire's best-kept secrets. This 76-mile circular walk has been designed to take in the best of the Wolds and keeps to the high ground where possible.

We completed this walk in four days and stayed in a cottage in the centre. The public transport and accommodation along the route is limited, therefore you will need to do some planning if you intend to do the entire circuit.

It is not particularly well known and does not have 'national trail' status, but it is a little hidden gem that is just waiting to be explored.

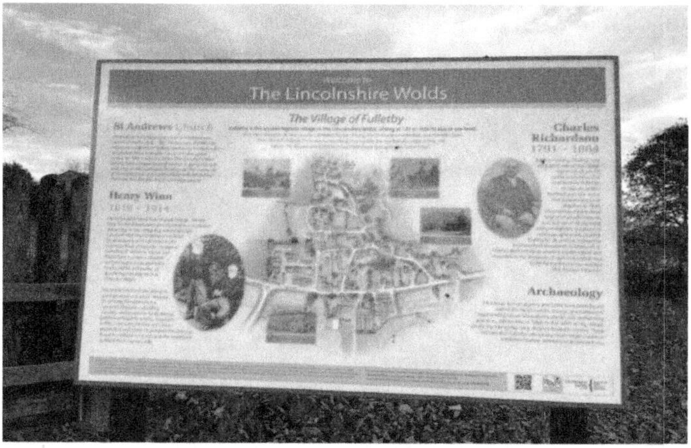

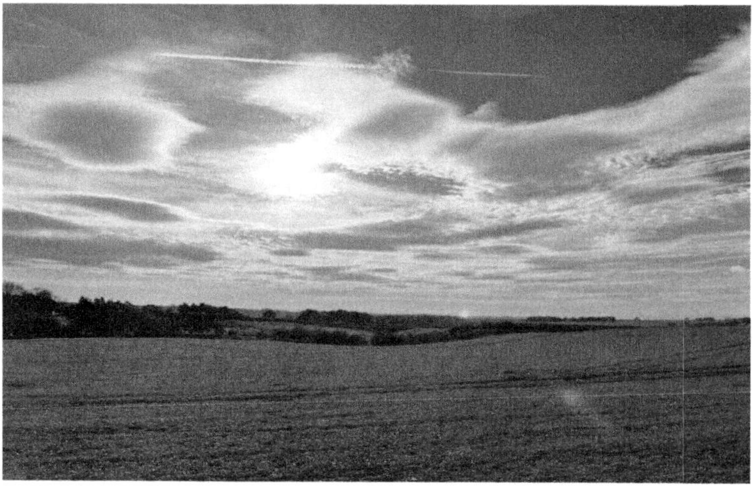

- WHITE CLIFFS TRAIL

The White Cliffs Trail was created in 1987 by Dover District Council to link the towns of Dover, Deal, and Sandwich, going along the famous 'white cliffs' to the east of Dover to Deal, with an inland return through the beautiful Kent countryside.

It is said to be 28 miles long – however, by my watch it was 31 miles.

It is a beautiful and diverse route taking in the clifftops, the coastline, the docks of Dover, and the remote countryside and villages.

At the time, we were on a family holiday and the path passed by the end of our garden, which made the logistics of the start/finish very easy – really, it would have been rude not to do it!

There is one section running alongside a dyke, which was probably the most challenging as it was approx. 8ft high in brambles and overgrowth and was obviously not well-walked.

Picking my way through that, with dykes either side, for approx. two miles was a bit daunting to say the least. Other than that, it's a pleasant good day's hike with plenty of places to stop for refreshments and scenic photo opportunities.

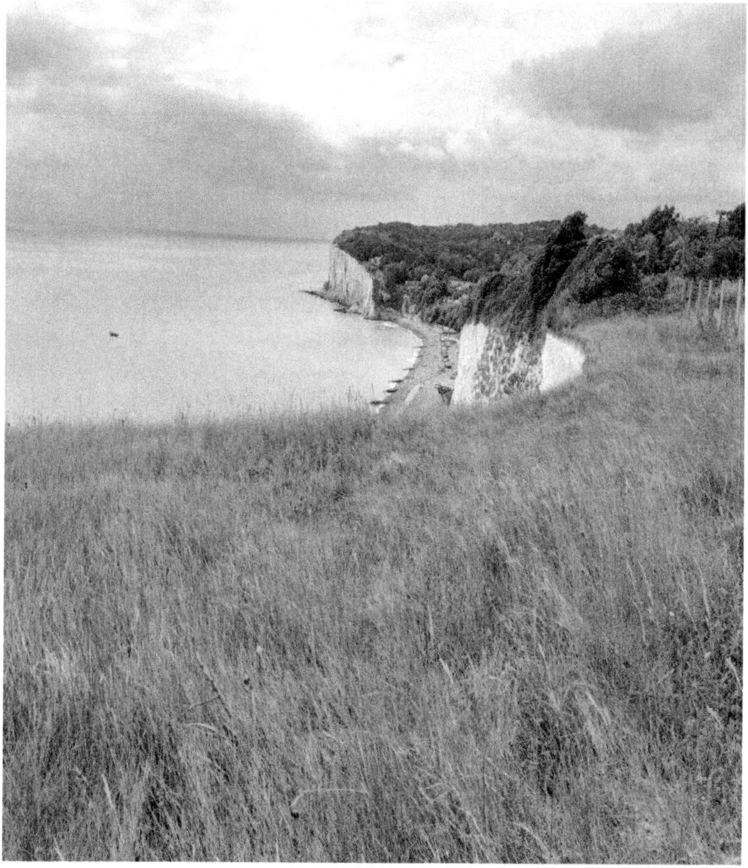

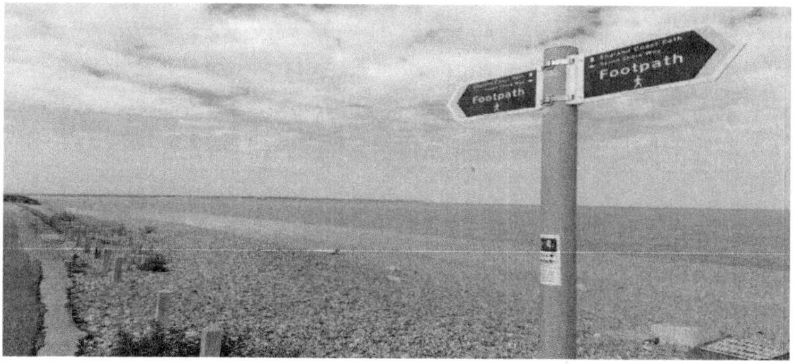
Footpath
Footpath

- EVEREST BASE CAMP (NEPAL)

The trek to Base Camp begins in the town of Lukla in the Solukhumbu region of Nepal. To access this town from Kathmandu involves turning your life over to a trusted pilot and boarding a tiny plane that is set to land on one of the world's shortest runways.

This trek can be done in various time periods, but we took an 11-day trip that was eight days up and three days down.

You don't have to be a mountaineer to manage this, but you do need a good level of fitness – and be prepared to experience symptoms of altitude sickness. Base Camp is situated at 5364m (the summit being 8848m) so altitude adjustment is definitely required.

The accommodation mostly consists of tea houses, which are basic but cute. Hot water is scarce and, as you increase in height, so is palatable food. The food is basic (pasta, pancakes, omelettes etc.) but it does the job. Having plentiful fluid is vital, and hot lemon with ginger is great to take the edge off the sickness. Alcohol is strictly off the menu until you return to Kathmandu.

This was one of my most amazing experiences. Seeing the world's tallest mountain in such close proximity, and hiking through some of the most basic yet beautiful villages, was a real privilege.

We had Sherpas (and yaks) carrying our camp up the mountain for us. These Sherpas are true human champions, with many of them skipping up the mountain with little more than flip flops on their feet. I was in total awe.

I think the part that sticks out as most memorable for me was the final day's hike into Base Camp itself, through the Khumbu region. It was more than cold, the air was thin and dry, and it was the most beautiful yet inhospitable place I've ever been. This is where we all seemed to contract the dreaded Khumbu cough (though luckily, not until we returned to Kathmandu).

The day before this, between Lobuche and Gorak Shep, we went through Chukla Lare, which is an area hosting memorials of all the brave mountaineers who have lost their lives while summiting the Everest Peak. The famous American mountaineer Scott Fischer, who lost his life in 1996, is amongst them. This was truly a humbling (albeit a little eerie) place to be.

The nights were well below zero degrees, and all water bottles and liquids were frozen (this was inside the tea houses).

The thing that will remain stamped on my memory for not-so-pleasant reasons is the powder room facilities... rancid... rancid... rancid... no more need be said.

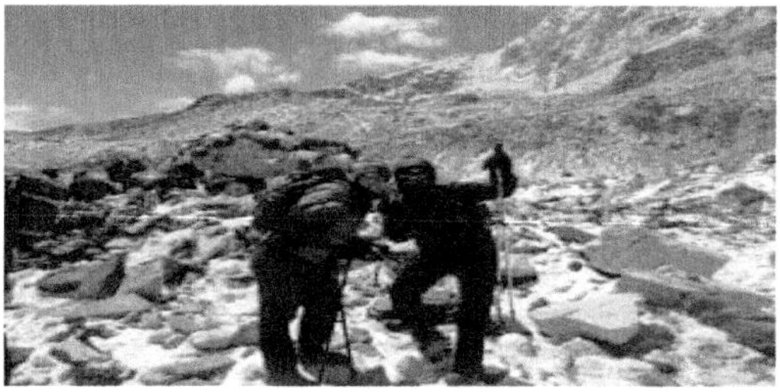

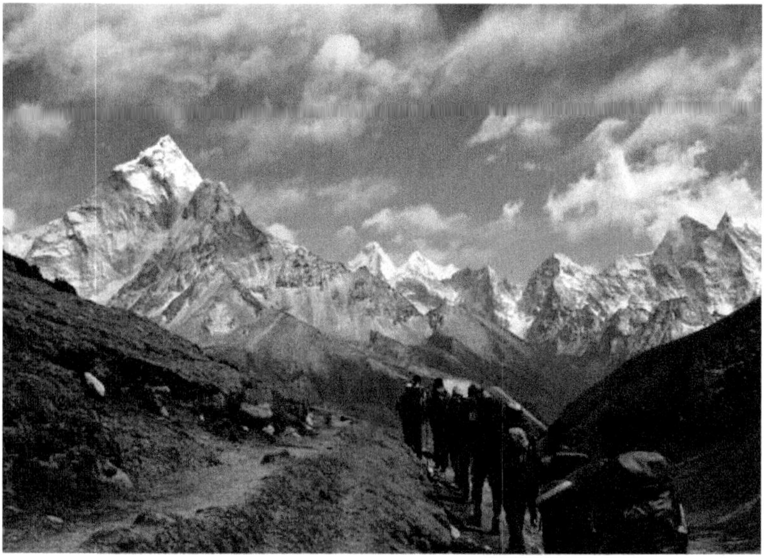

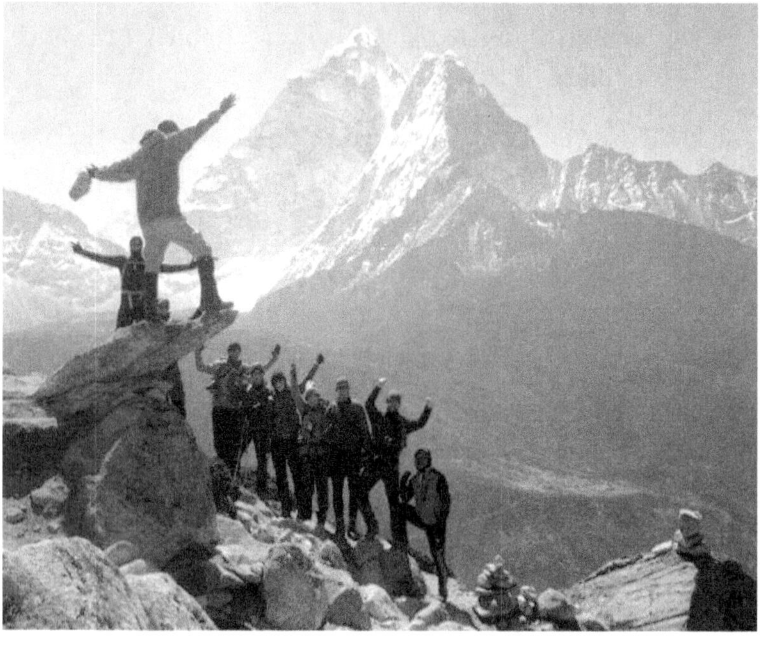

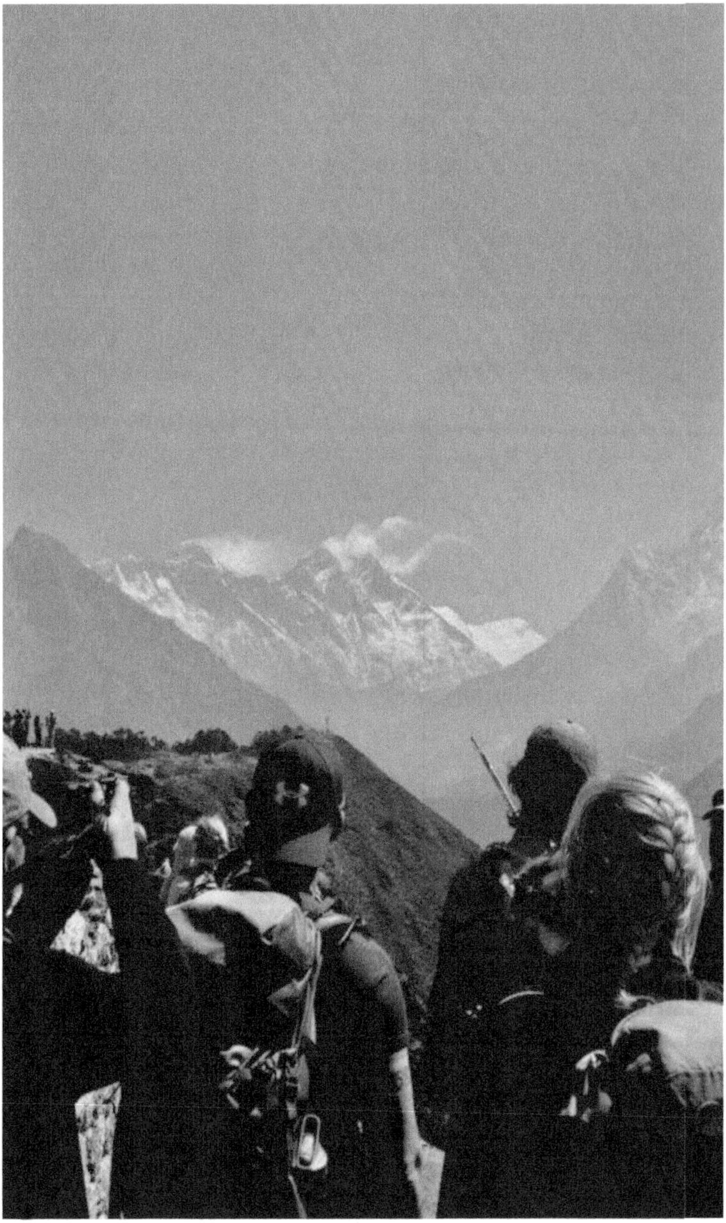

- INCA TRAIL (PERU)

The Inca Trail is a well-established four-day, three-night hike leading from the town of Ollantaytambo in Peru all the way to Machu Picchu via the iconic Sun Gate. It may only be approx. 25 miles… however, most of these miles are up steep, narrow Andean mountain paths at altitude.

You need to have a certain level of fitness for this one due to the steep inclines and the altitude issues you may or may not suffer from. I suffered initially with this, but I went with an organised group and they acclimatised us slowly in order for us to adapt.

Of course, arriving at the Sun Gate for sunrise and seeing the spectacular Machu Picchu from a height is no doubt the highlight of the trip. It is a beautiful, magical, spiritual place, and it's no wonder that it's classed as one of the New Seven Wonders of the World.

I did this trek in 2018 as part of a group. We had porters that carried our gear and set up camp ahead of our arrival each night. They cooked our meals, heated us water each morning for washing, and packed up camp daily to move onto the next destination. They would storm past us (although we would leave before them in the mornings) and our camp would be all set up by the time we arrived. They are the absolute heroes of these excursions; it would be very difficult to hike the trail without their care, knowledge, and support.

When it comes to this sort of challenge, the group of people you hike with is a game changer in terms of your experience. I've been blessed to have met – and am so very privileged to have walked with – some of the most amazing and inspirational human beings.

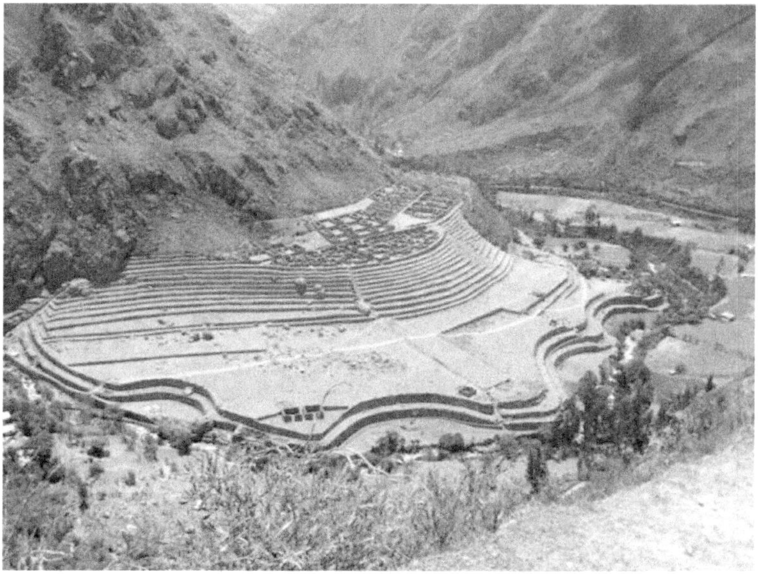

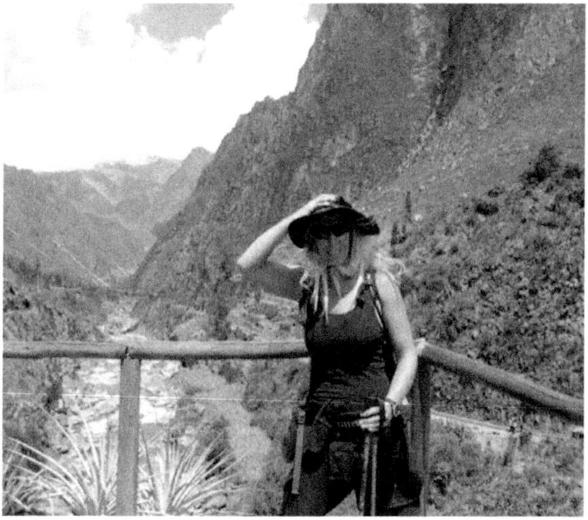

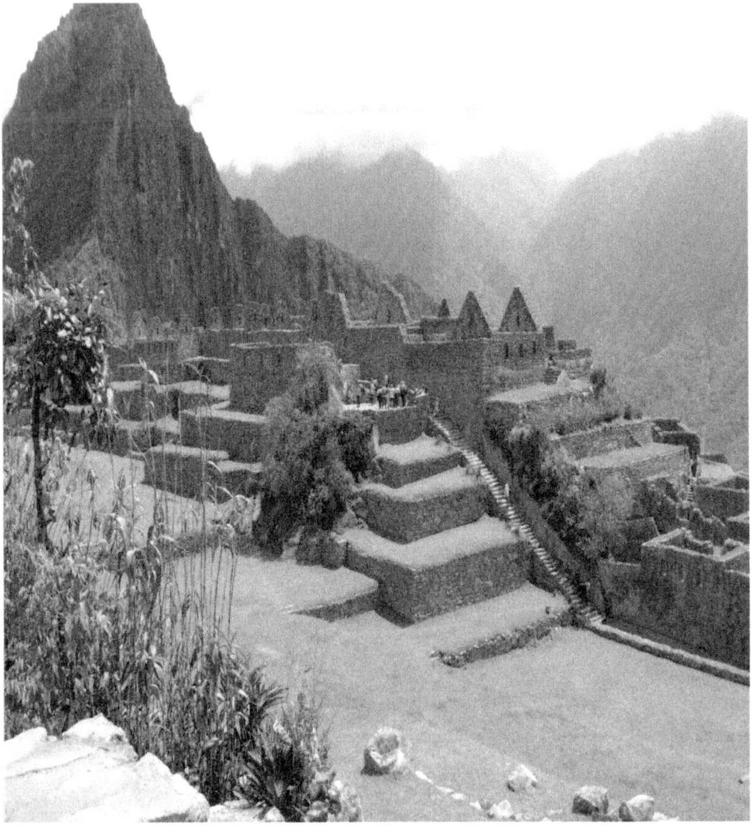

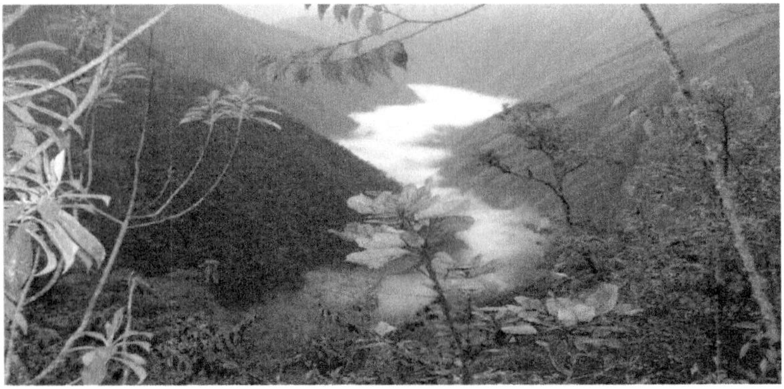

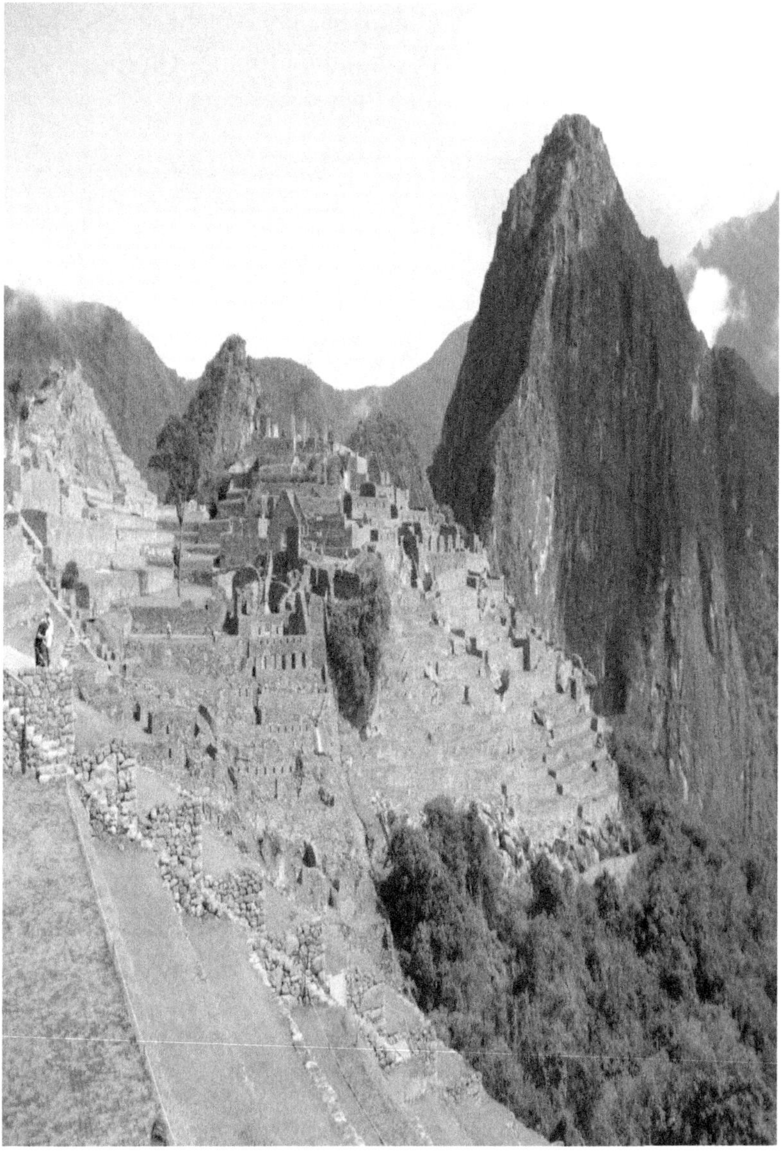

- KILIMANJARO (TANZANIA)

At 5895 metres, Mount Kilimanjaro is the highest mountain in Africa and the tallest freestanding mountain in the world. It is one of the famous Seven Summits.

I did this walk on the Machame route in 2019 with an organised group with 10 others. It was an eight-day trek (six days up and two days down).

The terrain on Kilimanjaro varies, covering around 38 miles and ascending from 2000m to 5895m and back down. The Machame route passes through cultivated farmland, forests, and alpine heath, across a lunar-like volcanic desert and up to a glaciated summit. It is not a technical climb – no rock climbing or specialist equipment needed – but it is high!
The weather and temperature can vary dramatically. The paths are in good condition and are well-trodden. There are some steep sections though, like the great Barranco Wall, which is in fact a scramble.

Due to the increase in altitude, the higher you go the more difficult it becomes, and it really can take its toll on your body.

We camped, with the porters carrying our camp and gear on ahead for us each day. They are just super human!

Summiting this peak was the hardest thing I have ever achieved. By the time we reached summit night I'd had very little sleep, and I also had a stomach bug and had lost my appetite completely. This caused fatigue, weakness, and dehydration, not to mention the issues with toileting!

Even to this day, I don't know how I got to the top of that mountain. I do, however, recall hallucinating, sleepwalking, and being force-fed jelly beans by my guide.

When we reached the summit, the sunrise – with the clouds beneath us – was truly out of this world, and just about made up (I think!) for the effort it took to get there.

This was a bittersweet experience for me. My friend Cheryl joined me on this trip. Sadly, she suffered with severe altitude sickness early on in the climb and, shockingly and devastatingly, she passed away on the mountainside. This rocked us all but, as a group, we decided to continue to the top; that was what we'd all gone there for, and I felt sure it was what Cheryl would have wanted us to do.

I was lucky enough to have booked some days off after the summit to head to the island of Zanzibar. I needed this time to recoup and reflect, and to process all that had happened in the previous days. Needless to say that despite achieving the summiting, and sharing this experience with the most supportive and beautiful of people, this is not somewhere I'll be rushing back to anytime soon.

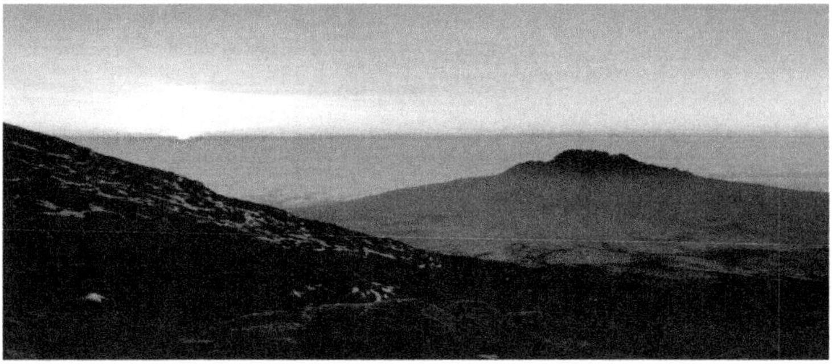

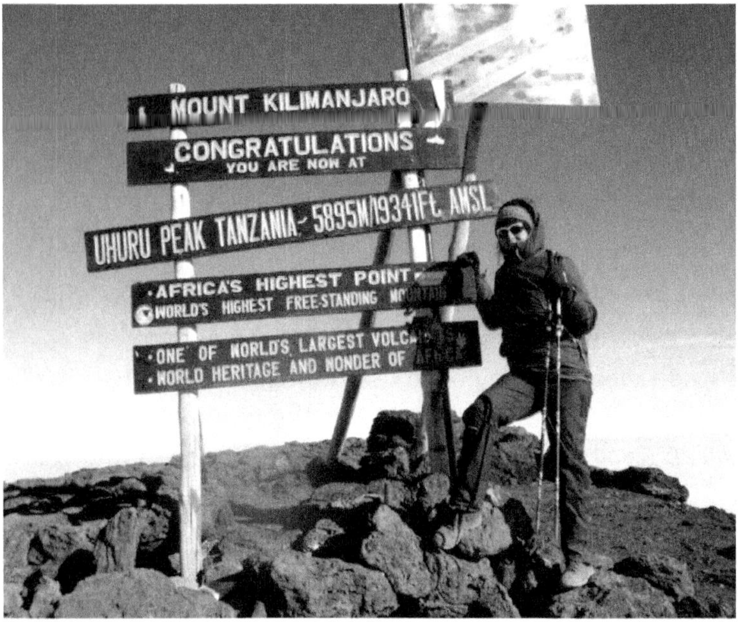
MOUNT KILIMANJARO
CONGRATULATIONS
YOU ARE NOW AT
UHURU PEAK TANZANIA - 5895M/19341Ft. AMSL
AFRICA'S HIGHEST POINT
WORLD'S HIGHEST FREE-STANDING
ONE OF WORLD'S LARGEST
WORLD HERITAGE AND WONDER OF

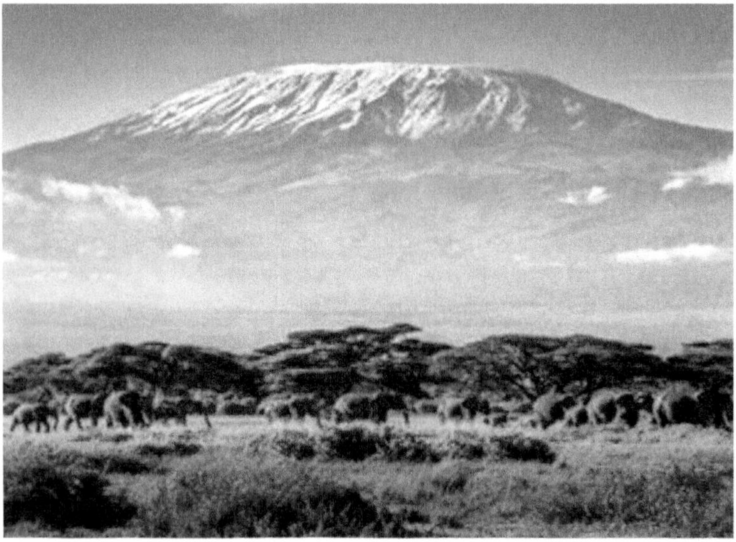

- ATLAS MOUNTAINS (MOROCCO)

The Atlas Mountains are a mountain range in Morocco, North Africa that separate the Sahara Desert from the Mediterranean Sea and the Atlantic Ocean. The range's highest peak is Toubkal with an elevation of 4167m.

This was just a day's hike in 2019 with some friends and a private guide whilst on a Pilates holiday in Morocco. As you would expect of a day's hike of this mountain, it was hot, dry, and dusty. Our guide was local and lived on the mountain itself. He was very knowledgeable and brought us to a beautiful restaurant near his local village for a tagine lunch. A day's hike is obviously not going to take you very high, but it was enough to experience some of the mountain villages and their ways of life.

It's definitely somewhere I would like to explore further or do a longer trek of at some point in the future.

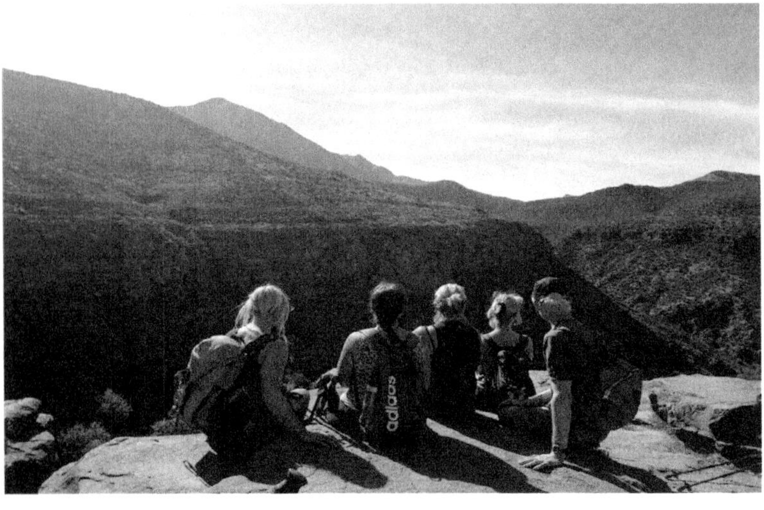

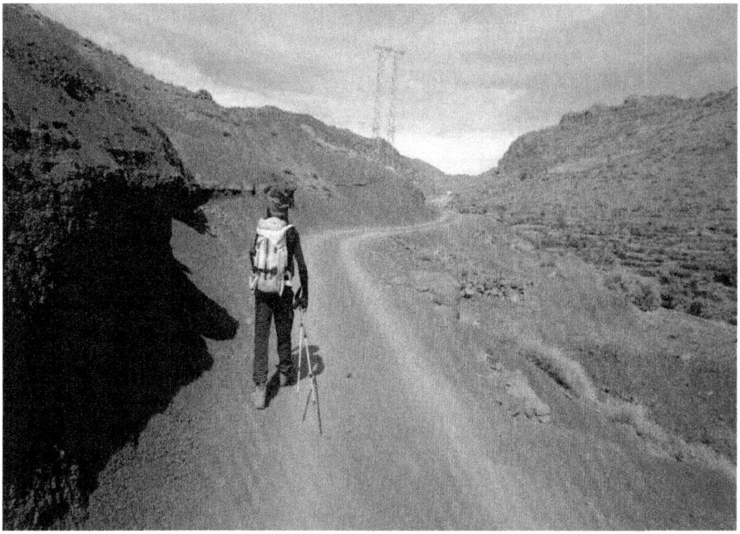

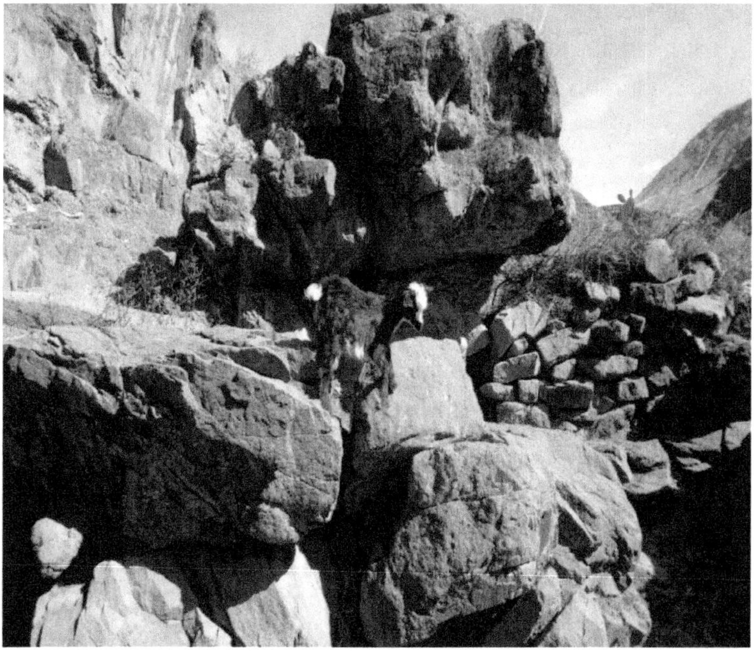

- THE CAMINO DE SANTIAGO

The Camino de Santiago is a network of ancient pilgrim routes across Europe which started in the 9th century and is walked by thousands of people each year. All routes meet at the end point being the tomb of St. James in Santiago in north-west Spain.

The route we took was the Camino Francés which stretches nearly 800 km from St. Jean-Pied-du-Port near Biarritz in France to Santiago. We only hiked the last 100 km of this trail from Sarria into Santiago over approx. 5 days.

It is not a quiet route by any means. It was rare to find any section of the trail where there were no other hikers. It was very peaceful though and a strong sense of unity with everyone you meet moving in the same direction to the same destination point.

I was not expecting it to be as green and lush as it was and it is not dissimilar to parts of the UK. Including a couple of days of rain.

There are copious amounts of cafes and albergues all along the trail so access to food ,drink and toilet facilities are plentiful.

Traditionally pilgrims would stay in hostels or shared accommodations. (We cheated and used hotels.)

It is nearly impossible to get lost on this trail. There are regular markers and the famous shell symbols can be found frequently, pointing you in the right direction.

This walk would be very safe and easy to do as a solo hiker. Especially if you are starting out and new to solo walking.

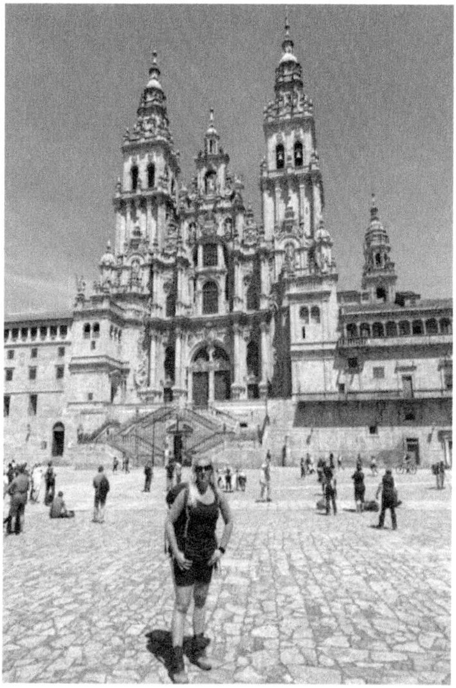

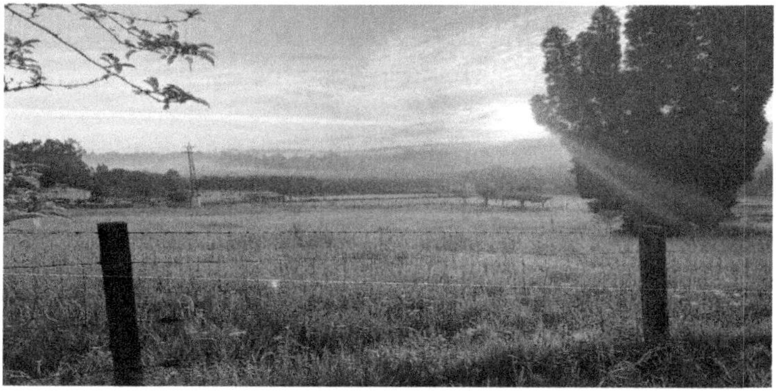

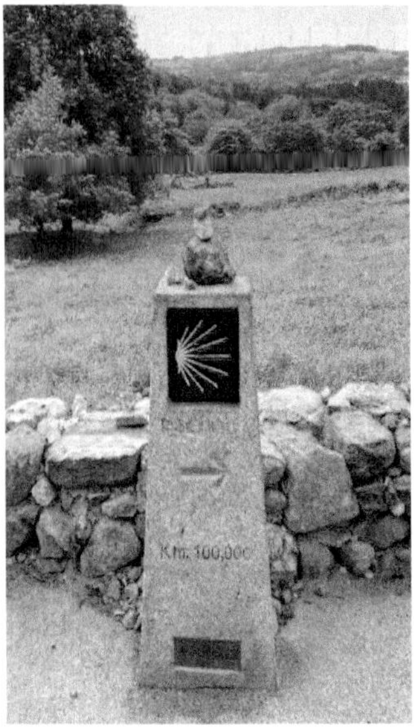

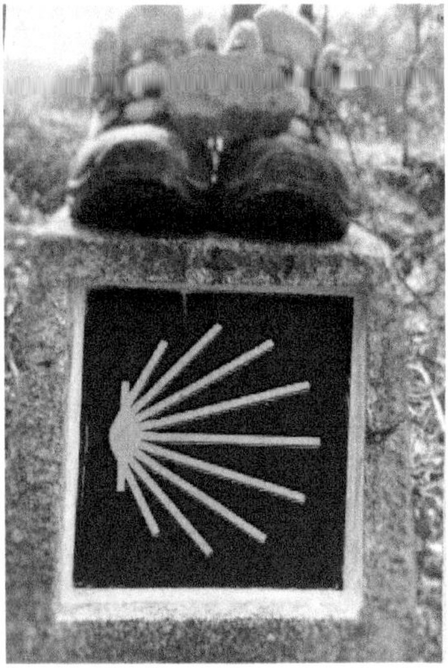

- TO BE CONTINUED…

I have many more adventures just waiting to be accomplished. My list never actually decreases because, when I'm out hiking or hearing other people's intrepid stories, I learn about all the other places out there that are simply waiting to be explored. I become intrigued, get a tingle down my spine and a twinkle in my eye, and on the list they go.

Walking makes me feel alive. It makes me feel connected to the earth beneath me and to my own mind, body, and soul. As long as I'm blessed enough to be able to do so, I shall keep on walking…

ACKNOWLEDGEMENTS

At the time of writing this book, I was in quite a dark and difficult place in my life. I never stopped getting out there and being with nature, but certain circumstances made this more difficult for me, both physically and mentally.

Writing this book has been my therapy. It has kept me focused on something I have a true passion for, and through my writing I have been able to relive all the amazing journeys, wonderful adventures, and incredible experiences I am so thankful to have experienced.

This book has made me feel immensely proud of myself. It has highlighted all I've achieved so far in my life and made me think hard about all I have left to give to this world, to myself, and to others.

I want to thank my very dear friend Catherine, who inspired me to put all my adventures down on paper. She has always been so encouraging of what I do, she has joined me on some of these wonderful trips, and she will always be a rock to me. She is also my best and most crazy party companion!

I would also like to thank my sisters, my earth angels who have shared my journey of loss and grief in losing our parents, but in doing so we have become each other's pillars in life. I am so truly privileged to have these two shining stars beside me in all I do.

All those fellow hikers and explorers whom I've been blessed to walk beside, I admire and respect every one of you and am so honoured to have had your company, to share the smiles and the tears and to have been a part of your own personal journeys. There are far too many to mention individually, but each one of you has played a part in my story so far – and, without you, I may never have accomplished my goals.

If this book reaches only one person and empowers them to go and achieve everything they've been dreaming of but have never felt able to do alone, then my work here is done.

REFERENCES/FURTHER READING

- Andrews K (London 2020) Wanderers, A History Of Women Walking, *Reaktion Books.*

- Armitage S (2012) Walking Home*, Faber and Faber*

- Blyton E (1951) The Faraway Tree*, Newnes*

- Gilbert E (2006) Eat, Pray, Love*, Penguin Publishing UK*

- Lewis SA (London 2018) The Girl Outdoors, *Bloomsbury Publishing UK*

- Ransome A (1930) Swallows & Amazons, *Jonathon Cape*

- Strayed C (2012) Wild, *Knopf*

- https://en.wikipedia.org

- Winn R (2018) The Salt path, *Penguin Publishing UK*

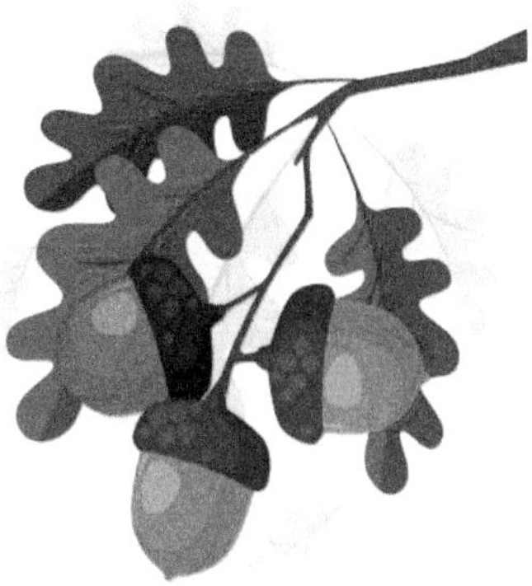

AUTHOR

Louise Akern

Publisher: Kindle Direct Publishing
https://kdp.amazon.com/en (2023) 1st Edition

Printed in Great Britain
by Amazon

21143861R00068